CW00550252

The Complete HAPPY Dachshund Guide

Raise a Happy, Well-Mannered Dog and Avoid Dog Behavior Professionals for Life

- Dog Happiness Tips
- Techniques for a Well-behaved Dachshund
- Prevent Behavior Issues
- Fulfill Your Puppy's Needs
- Be the Ideal Guardian
- Avoid Common Mistakes

Asia Moore

Dog Behavior Expert & Acclaimed Author

Copyrighted © 2020

Author: Asia Moore
www.K-9SuperHeroesDogWhispering.com
www.KnowsToNose.com
www.MustHavePublishing.com
www.askboris.com

Editor & Researcher: Alex Warrington, Ph.D.

Published by:
Worldwide Information Publishing
London
Great Britain
2020

ALL RIGHTS RESERVED. This book contains material protected under International and Federal Copyright Laws and Treaties.

Any unauthorized reprint or use of this material is strictly prohibited. No part of this book may be reproduced or transmitted in any form or by any means, electronic, mechanical or otherwise, including photocopying or recording, or by any information storage and retrieval system without express written permission from the author.

"Dogs are small rays of light caught on the Earth a short time to brighten our days."
— Unknown

Preface

It takes time, commitment, tenacity, consistency and knowledge to raise a happy and healthy Dachshund that doesn't suffer from health and behavioral issues.

This book is NOT like most other breed-specific books, because we believe that it's far better for all parties concerned (human and canine) to **prevent** problems rather than suffering the frustrations of living with or learning how to eliminate problems and rehabilitate a dog that has already developed health or behavioral issues.

It is always better to prevent unwanted behaviors than to hope you, or someone else, may have what it takes to eliminate them in the future, after your family is at their wits end, your neighbors hate you, your friends no longer visit, your dog has been deemed dangerous, and you're having guilty thoughts of re-homing every time you drive past your local SPCA.

If you want a happy, well-mannered Dachshund canine companion to be a loyal, valued member of your family, it absolutely matters how you raise your dog.

Every breed has uniquely different needs. Even those that were once working breeds that are now companion breeds.

For instance, a Border Collie is a very smart, high-energy dog that excels at the job of sheep herding. Therefore, if you expect this dog to sit around doing nothing all day while you're at work, you will most likely return to holes in your drywall, torn apart couches and a home that looks like it's been through a cyclone.

On the other hand, the Shih Tzu lap dog, which was originally only permitted to be owned by royalty, sat on silk pillows, was used to warm beds, has vastly different daily exercise requirements, and would be a poor choice for someone requiring a companion that could protect them from being mugged on streets ravaged by gang warfare.

The charming and tenacious Dachshund is a small-sized breed of hound that was originally used for hunting. Learning the basics about this breed will help you to determine if this is the right dog for you and your family.

Every dog breed has different talents and needs and when you decide to share your life with a particular breed, if you want a happy and well-adjusted companion, you must also be prepared to provide your dog with what he or she needs to be a happy member of your family.

Almost all canine problems, both mentally and physically, are a direct result of ignorance or unwillingness on the part of the human guardian to choose the right dog for their particular energy and lifestyle. It takes research, time and commitment to learn what each dog truly needs.

This book is uniquely different, and humans reading it need to clearly understand that the pages of this book are not all about describing what to do to eliminate problematic canine behaviors that have already occurred.

Rather, the main focus of this breed-specific book is to describe what the human guardian needs to understand and commit to doing on a daily basis in order to match the Dachshund's needs, so that they can raise a happy, healthy and well-behaved dog that never has to experience behavioral issues.

Do not expect this book to be like all the others that set out endless correlations between specific mal-behaviors and what steps or actions the human guardian can take in an attempt to correct them.

In other words, this book is a totally new slant on raising a happy and healthy Dachshund, because the main focus here is on the <u>prevention</u> of behavioral issues rather than addressing them after they have already surfaced.

About the Author

Asia Moore

Dog Behavior Expert & Acclaimed Author

Ever since my first birthday, I was immersed in nature, and have always enjoyed a special connection with all creatures, both great and small. I learned to communicate and "talk" with many animals in their language, both wild and domesticated. At approximately the age of twelve, dogs began to become the main focus of my life, when I set about training and grooming my first puppy.

When friends and neighbors began to recognize how well behaved my dog was, and were subsequently impressed with all the tricks and routines she could perform, often without a spoken word, they asked me to train their dogs, too.

I've been so fortunate to have experienced the unconditional love of so many dogs over the years, all of who taught me many different life lessons. I began this journey with my first mixed breed ("Cindy") who protected me from my marauding brothers, then my mixed breed ("Pepper") who had an amazing human vocabulary and always knew when someone was not to be trusted, my Blue Heeler ("Bugsy") who would hike endless trails and swim miles with me, to my current loving Shih Tzu ("Boris") and all my clients' dogs in between.

Now, some 40 years later, and endless different breeds, including these patient and affectionate clowns of the dog world, and many hybrids and mutts, from tiny Chihuahuas to bouncing Belgians, a cascade of fur friends have passed through my life.

For the last 40 years, I have been managing my dog whispering, dog sitting and grooming businesses and have enjoyed countless experiences of working with dogs of all breeds and their guardians. It hasn't always been easy, and while I've had my fair share of struggles and setbacks, I've always loved and been passionate about what I do.

All these years of experience taught me invaluable lessons in all aspects of the human-canine relationship interaction. For instance, I learned how to effectively communicate with our canine friends, understand their needs and help them and their guardians lead a fulfilling and happy life together. *What could be better than that?*

Clients' dogs now remain the focal point of my dog whispering, sitting and grooming life, while I also focus on writing children's books and breed-specific books. I have so far authored over 300 dog breed books, where my goal is to pass on my knowledge and experience to all responsible dog owners (**Must Have Publishing.com**). At the same time, I continue to train human guardians, so that they can improve their relationships with their dogs and understand how to prevent and alleviate behavioral issues (**K-9 Super Heroes Dog Whispering.com**).

As well, I have recently added an additional online branch to my business, which I call "Knows To Nose" to help humans "know" how to choose the right dog "nose" for their energy and lifestyle, before they make the wrong decision and end up with troubling problems.

I am also often called upon to speak to groups about the changing roles for the canine population and how they now fit into our modern world. As well, I help humans and their chosen canines establish harmonious relationships with neighbors for those residing in multi-family living situations, such as apartment and condominium complexes.

I feel blessed that the canine world has been a major part of my life for so many years, as it never gets old. I continuously stay in touch with my clients through my business websites and personal consultations and I love how there is always room to learn more, because every unique dog brings new lessons to light and enhances everyone's life in untold, indescribable ways.

I'd like to thank you for purchasing "The Complete Happy Dachshund Guide" and reassure you that the pages of this book contain the distilled knowledge of over 40 years experience, which, by the way, includes helping a Dachshund suffering from anxiety about crossing over unfamiliar, slippery floor tiles.

When taken to heart, the knowledge, tips and techniques in this book can help you along your special journey inside the amazing world of our canine friends, so that you can know the unconditional love, special bond and joy that only our four-legged companions selflessly offer to us flawed humans.

Visit Asia online at the following locations:

www.K-9SuperHeroesDogWhispering.com
www.KnowsToNose.com
www.MustHavePublishing.com
www.askboris.com

Table of Contents

Chapter 1: Introduction

*"Properly trained, a man
can be dog's best friend."*
— Corey Ford

The purpose of this book is to focus on the important steps the humans in this relationship really need to be aware of and commit to providing in order to ensure that their Dachshund companion can live a happy and healthy life, which in turn will ensure a happy relationship for everyone.

Even though humans and dogs have been relying on one another for more than 30,000 years, it's still highly important that you take an honest look at your life, decide whether sharing your life with a dog is truly feasible, and then if it is, choose the companion that is best suited to your particular lifestyle.

Within the pages of this book you will find information to help you choose wisely by providing you with a clear understanding concerning whether or not YOU have what it takes to be the right match for raising a happy and well-mannered Dachshund companion.

In addition, this book describes in detail what the human guardian needs to keep in mind and commit to doing on a daily basis in order to match this charming companion's needs, so that they can raise a happy, healthy and well-behaved dog that never has to experience behavioral issues.

All the information, suggestions, tips and advice given in this publication is the result of more than 40 years experience helping humans positively and effectively interact with the canine world.

If you take all that is written on these pages to heart, and regularly and consistently apply them, your friendly and curious Dachshund will be a happy family member that will not have to suffer from any behavioral problems. In other words, the focus is placed on prevention, rather than trying to correct any issues after they have surfaced.

Every Chapter of this book contains valuable information that will provide you with a solid understanding of the breed and the steps you need to take to raise a happy and well-behaved dog.

For instance, **Chapter 2** – *"Asia's Happiness Tips"* sets out a summary of what she personally believes makes for a happy Dachshund and encourages you to ask yourself what YOU think would make this dog happy.

Chapter 3 – *"Overview of the Happy Dachshund"* will outline vital statistics, coat colors and common features, intelligence, temperament and interesting secrets and facts that may not be commonly known. In order to raise a contented dog, you need to have some basic knowledge of the history of the Dachshund breed, to help you choose wisely so that you are able to comprehend this dog's needs.

Chapter 4 – *"Healthy Dachshund = Happy Dog"* is where you will find out what you need to know about medical care, safety and health issues that may affect this toy-sized breed, including common diseases and viruses, allergies and canine CPR procedures that could save a life. Needless to say, if your dog is not physically healthy, he or she will not be a happy canine companion for very long, because suffering from health-related issues will undoubtedly create a miserable and ill-mannered dog.

In **Chapter 5** – *"Let Your Dog BE a Happy Dog"*, you will find information about how to let your Dachshund actually BE a dog, rather than attempting to turn them into a fur human, which can make for a very confused, unhappy and ill-mannered canine.

Chapter 6 – *"Every Happy Dachshund Wants Exercise"*, first outlines some of the original history of this purebred dog that has become a companion; if you know what they were bred to do, you will better understand how important it is to commit to the daily exercise routines recommended in this book, without which your dog will not be happy for very long.

Chapter 7 – *"Feeding the Happy Dachshund"*, is where you will find information about the structure of the canine jaw, various food options and feeding suggestions as well as treats to avoid for raising a happy and healthy companion.

In **Chapter 8** – *"Care of the Happy Dachshund"*, you will find travel safety tips, licensing, insurance, essential grooming procedures and important care of nails, ears, teeth and paws, all of which will help you to raise a happy dog.

While this information might seem generic, imagine how you might feel going for months without washing your hair, cutting your nails or brushing your teeth. Unfortunately, that is the reality for many dogs, because their owners have not been properly advised with respect to the importance of good grooming habits. How happy and well behaved do you think such a poorly cared for Dachshund would be?

Chapter 9 – *"Are YOU the Ideal Happy Dachshund Guardian?"* is concerned with asking yourself some serious questions, including whether your energy, activity, commitment and lifestyle matches what this dog needs to be happy and well behaved. It's vital for you to give serious consideration to these questions when considering this breed, because should you choose the wrong dog to share your life with, everybody will be miserable.

Chapter 10 – *"Humans Make a LOT of Stupid Mistakes"* outlines that far too often we humans, without even realizing it, are the cause of creating behavioral problems in our canine companions. You will find out what are some of the common mistakes to avoid (and the right thing to do!) when it comes to socialization, accidental rewards, fear of noises, the right collars, basic rules and boundaries, adolescent craziness and more.

Simply being aware of the many mistakes we humans can often inadvertently be guilty of when raising our canine companions, can mean the difference between a Happy Dachshund with no behavioral issues or a life of frustration and correction.

Chapter 11 – *"Happy Dachshund Body Language"*, outlines the basics of learning canine body language, and will help you be safe around other dogs. Learning to properly "read" a dog's intentions can prevent an unwanted encounter with another canine or human, and this will help to ensure that everyone remains safe and happy.

In Chapter 12 – *"Training Basics for a Happy Dachshund"*, you will learn valuable training tips and routines that will help to keep your dog truly happy and well behaved for their entire life. It's no surprise that a properly trained companion will be a much happier companion that everyone enjoys being around, and will be far less likely to develop behaviour issues later in life.

Developing a basic training program and learning to teach your dog commands and discipline is all part of starting your dog off on the right paw.

Chapter 13 – *"What If You Slip Up?"* is only necessary because we humans tend to get too busy and overwhelmed with the rigors of daily living, which means we sometimes forget to be consistent with providing what our particular dog may need to be happy. If you slip up, this Chapter has outlined a few of the more common behavioral issues and how to quickly get yourself back on track.

Chapter 14 – *"Surprise Bonus Chapter"* is a Question and Answer section containing a few human/canine situations, with humans asking questions and wise words from the perspective of the dog, which answers the questions. You will also find an amusing and educational true story about a happy dog that just refused to set one paw on the newly installed tiles in his family home.

Take heed humans, because when you honestly assess your own compatibility, lifestyle and energy level for being the right guardian for the Dachshund, and are vigilant about following the advice and tips outlined in the following pages, you can raise a healthy and happy dog that will be a joy to live with and will never have to suffer from any behavioral issues.

Chapter 2: Asia's Happiness Tips

"Dogs do speak, but only to those who know how to listen."
— Orhan Pamuk

The following few paragraphs are a summary of my own personal ramblings, beliefs, and ideas about what I think makes for a happy Dachshund.

While I hope you may wholeheartedly agree, it's absolutely okay if you have other ideas, or if you may have an entirely different take on this subject, because we will all have our own "personal" ideas about what constitutes happiness for the amusing and entertaining Dachshund, and if your ideas are different from mine, this does not mean that they are any less valid.

If you're considering sharing your life with the clever and sometimes stubborn Dachshund, and have never before really sat down and consciously thought about what would make this particular breed truly happy, while you may gain a little insight from reading about my own personal beliefs, I encourage you to take the time to do this exercise yourself. If you have a family, get them involved in this fun exercise, too.

When you take the time to sit with a piece of paper and pen and begin to write down what YOU think makes a Dachshund happy, you may be surprised about what surfaces, and this simple exercise may inspire you and your family to discover new ways to bond with your dog, which will be the basis of having a truly happy relationship.

I'll help to get you started with the following question:
"What do you think would make a Dachshund happy?"

I've shared the last 14 years of my life with a wonderfully loving and well behaved Shih Tzu and I believe that the very best start you can make, with respect to "happiness" when first bringing home your new Dachshund puppy is to do all you can to reassure him or her that they are not alone (see below).

Happy New Surroundings

The puppy will be understandably nervous about the new and unfamiliar faces, surroundings and smells, and will be missing their mother, other siblings and everything in their environment they had grown used to during their first 8 to 10 weeks of life.

Make sure that you don't overwhelm your new puppy with too much all at once. For instance, close off rooms that you don't need access to and encourage your puppy to come to you as you wander about in a smaller space.

Happy Sleep Patterns

When it's time to go to bed, take your puppy outside for a bathroom break, and then make sure that you have a nice, cozy kennel all ready for your new puppy with a soft lining or blanket and place their new bedroom inside your room, so that they will be able to hear and see you.

__Unless you want your Dachshund to sleep on your bed (or IN your bed because these dogs like to burrow under blankets) when they're fully grown, even when they may have wet or dirty feet, or just rolled in a dead rat, now is the time to exercise a little tough love as the new puppy will most likely not want to be alone in their kennel and will prefer sleeping next to you or burrowed under the covers.__

If your bed is large enough to accommodate their kennel, this is the best way to help your puppy have a happy sleep time because they will be next to you, but still safe inside their own kennel, and as they grow larger they will be used to their kennel and will not mind that it is sitting on the floor. Congratulations! You've just created a routine that will ensure happy and respectful sleeping patterns for your dog.

Happy Puppy Play

Taking the time for regular play sessions with your new Dachshund puppy will certainly make them very happy, so make sure you set aside several times during your day when you stop with the human work and chores and engage your puppy in fun games for 5 or 10 minutes at least three or four times a day.

Every puppy and dog needs some time in their day where they can relax and play a fun game, and this is the beginning of trust and respect between you and your fur friend.

Happy Puppy Housetraining

One of the very first things your new Dachshund puppy needs to learn is where the bathroom is, and the more vigilant you are, the fewer "accidents" will occur, which will make both of you much happier.

I taught my Shih Tzu (Boris) to ring a little bell whenever he needed to

 go outside, which is a very valuable "trick" to teach. Just hang a loud ringing bell at the end of a ribbon, string or rope from the doorknob where you will always take your dog through to go outside for a bathroom break. Every time you take them out, go to the bell, lift their paw and knock it against the bell to make it ring. Say *"Good boy, or girl – go pee?"* Then immediately take them out through this door.

Learn to pay attention and understand your dog's body language, so that you can help teach them proper bathroom habits at a very young age. This is a smart dog and it should not be difficult to quickly train them that outside is where they need to go to get to their bathroom.

When they wake up in the morning, take them outside immediately. Twenty minutes after they have eaten a meal, take them outside to relieve themselves. After a play session or when they've had a big drink of water, or woken up from a nap, take them outside. After they've gone pee or number 2, immediately praise and reward them with a treat.

Yes, to do this right, you and your puppy will be spending a lot of time going outside, but once their bladder grows larger and stronger, the number of hours he or she can "hold" it will increase, and the number of times your dog will have to visit the great outdoor bathroom during each day will markedly decrease.

 Use this bathroom training time also as a way to create a strong bond between you and your dog and as their first lessons in leash training and reward training for doing what you ask; if you take the time to go out with them while they're on leash, it's easy to train your dog to "go" on command, and as they mature, you'll be very glad that you took the time to do this.

Happy Puppy Feeding

 It's not rocket science to understand that providing your puppy or dog with the best nutrition from the very first day you bring them home will lead to a healthier fur friend, which in turn, will lead to a feel-good, energetic and happy companion.

Be aware of the importance of what you feed your dog and commit to doing the best you can to keep your canine friend healthy and happy. Read labels and feed them only the highest-quality food, so they have the best opportunity for a long life.

While it's important to start your puppy off with the right food, it's just as important to continue to feed your adult dog the very best diet. Please refer to Chapter 7 (Feeding the Happy Dachshund), where you will read about types of food, appropriate treats and more.

Happy Socializing

 Socializing a new puppy is one of the most important steps you can take to ensure that your chosen companion lives a happy and stress-free life.

When you don't take the time to properly socialize your Dachshund puppy, and indeed, keep on socializing throughout their lifetime, you can actually create many behavioral issues; some of these can be so severe that your dog may be in danger of having their life prematurely shortened, or having to wear a muzzle every time they are in public, should they act out aggressively toward a human or other animal.

Many times, I've been called upon to help a human alleviate aggressive tendencies being displayed by their canine companion, and in pretty much every instance, this could have been entirely avoided if the dog had been properly trained and socialized.

In the case of the adorable Dachshund, this popular small dog may become overly suspicious of strangers if you do not take the time to ensure that they are well-socialized and taught rules and boundaries, beginning at a young age.

Further, because they are a small breed that is relatively easy to carry around (especially the miniature size), if you make the mistake of coddling and babying this companion, you can end up creating an insecure dog, or worse, one that is downright disagreeable. Be careful not to create a dog that has a reputation for being an *"armpit alligator"* should anyone get too close.

When considering this breed, you should be aware that Dachshunds are statistically more aggressive to both strangers and other dogs. What might surprise many is that this cute and comical looking small breed has made it into the top ten breeds of *"Most Aggressive Dogs"*, or *"Dogs That Bite the Most"* on more than one occasion. More than 20% display aggressive tendencies that include biting other dogs, strangers and their owners, too.

When you consider this breed's hunting history and the fact that they were created to pursue badgers, which are quite vicious, it's no surprise that the fearless and tenacious Dachshund has the propensity for becoming aggressive.

Every dog must have a leader. While the charming, loving and playful Dachshund is a small size, they usually have a big personality and a feisty temperament. This is a small dog that can easily become stubborn and irritable if you push them too hard or too far and they will not hesitate to fight back if they believe they are being harshly treated.

Although charming, playful and very entertaining, this is a hunting breed with strong prey drive well known for their speed and quick reflexes when prey is within their sight.

 Be vigilant, because this is a dog that can escape out the door in a second to chase down a squirrel, a bird or the

neighbor's unlucky cat without a thought to crossing a busy street.

When not properly socialized, trained and taught to respect the word of their human guardians, even this small companion may be forced to take over the family "pack" and make human decisions. Unfortunately, this can get them and you into all sorts of unwanted troubles, especially should they decide to act out in an aggressive manner.

Any sort of aggression is a huge stress on both dog and human and, as we are all aware, stress shortens lives and prevents anyone from experiencing happiness, so help make your dog happy and make sure that you don't place the very heavy burden of making human decisions on the shoulders of your tiny canine companion.

While early socialization of a puppy is very important, keep in mind that it's just as important to continue your adult dog's socialization throughout their lifetime. Please refer to Chapter 10 (Humans Make a LOT of Stupid Mistakes) that outlines the many aspects of socializing your Dachshund.

Happy Training

Almost as important as proper socializing to keep your dog happy, is proper training, which should never be overlooked, unless you want to create an unstable Dachshund that barks and growls at everything and thinks they are the boss of all they survey.

This is a dog that will chase down a ball with **great** determination and ferocity as small things that move quickly excite and attract them and they will instantly snap into hunter mode.

 Most Dachshunds love to dig holes and enjoy tunneling in the ground and underneath the blankets and many are known to be excessive barkers.

Also, the Dachshund does not like to go outside when it's cold or wet, therefore, house training will go much more smoothly if you have a covered yard or train them to use an indoor potty station.

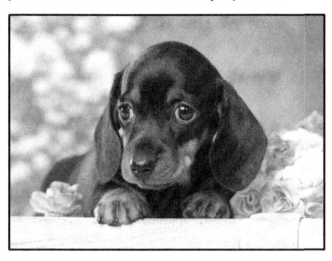

Don't be fooled by their smaller stature, because in order to keep any dog happy, they need to have both their body regularly exercised and their brain regularly challenged.

Start training this loyal and loving companion as soon as you bring him or her home from the breeder and you will have given yourself the best opportunity to have a happy, eager to comply and safe companion at your side before they are six months old. Of course, you will start out with very short training sessions of no more than a few minutes at a time, and as they slowly mature, you can increase the length of your sessions.

Make sure any training is a fun and happy time for both you and your dog, with lots of happy praise and treats, and he or she will quickly learn to trust and respect you as their leader and be eager for their next session.

While this puppy can begin training at an early age, when you continue their training throughout their life, this smart and affectionate companion will usually be an eager participant that is entirely capable of learning many commands, tricks, and hand signals, as well as several canine sports. See more in Chapter 12 (Training Basics for a Happy Dachshund).

Happy Exercising

While the Dachshund is smart and can certainly excel with training and learning new routines, which is exercise as well, they also need some down time, or some time off from your vigilant supervision.

Just like us humans, who need time where they don't have to think about work, our dogs also need some free time where they can enjoy romping and playing with the family or exploring the local woodland paths, rolling in the grass or lazing in the warm sunshine, and just being a dog.

While the Dachshund can be a moderate to higher-energy dog, depending on their age, they can also be a much more active companion, with a lively and playful temperament that loves to chase and romp with other small dogs.

 Especially when they are puppies, always be vigilant when walking a miniature version of this fur friend any place

where there may be large birds of prey present. Owls, hawks or eagles may consider them a food source.

Of course, with a smaller dog, your supervision of playtime is always a must, because allowing a smaller dog to play with a bigger and much heavier dog can mean that your smaller Dachshund inadvertently gets injured. Supervision is even more important when your Dachshund is very young and still growing, as well as when he or she gets older and is not as spry as they once were.

There are always more dangers with a small dog, and as the Dachshund has a much longer body on those short legs, you need to especially protect them from spinal injuries. However, being overprotective and carrying them everywhere can cause this dog to become an insecure, nasty biter that mindlessly barks at everyone.

Yes, protect this smaller companion when necessary, but also teach them rules and boundaries. Don't get caught up in dressing them like a human infant, and let them be a dog that walks on their own four paws. Otherwise, you may end up creating a cute companion with a maniacal personality that everyone but you hates.

While every dog is different, with respect to how much exercise they might need, and how active <u>YOU</u> are will also have an effect, the Dachshund usually requires a moderate amount of daily exercise to keep them mentally healthy and physically fit. You can learn much more about the exercises that will keep this dog happy in Chapter 6 (Every Happy Dachshund Wants Exercise).

Happy Visits to the Vet

Even though you may be feeding the best food, properly exercising, socializing and training your dog to be a calm and obedient member of your family, you will also want to have at least yearly visits to your chosen veterinarian's office to make sure all is well.

Start taking your dog to the vet's office even when they don't have any reason to be there, other than to receive a treat and friendly greetings, so that they get used to the different smells and people who work there because when you do this, your dog will learn that visits to the vet's office can be a happy time.

While it's ideal to get your puppy used to visits to the vet's office when they are still young, there is much you can do throughout the life of your adult dog that will help to keep these visits to a minimum. Be sure to read Chapter 8 (Care of the Happy Dachshund) that outlines many things you can do to help ensure your dog remains as healthy as possible.

Back to the pen and paper exercise.

When you pay attention, and take the time to think about the many things you can do that will keep your dog happy, even more ideas will present themselves along the way, and you and your chosen canine companion will enjoy a long and happy life together. Take my word for it, and *do make the time for this fun exercise* because you will thank me later.

In a Nutshell

The above paragraphs are a short synopsis of what I think makes for a Happy Dachshund, and I'm sure you may have many more ideas to contribute to this list.

The following Chapters of this book contain much more detail concerning what every conscientious Dachshund guardian needs to commit to, on a daily basis, in order to ensure that the human family and the chosen canine companion have the best opportunity for living a long, happy and healthy life together without ever having to experience any unwanted behavioral issues.

The loyal little Dachshund is a comical clown that loves to play games and will become very attached to their family. So much so, that they believe it is their right to sleep under the bed covers in your bed.

When you want to raise a Happy Dachshund canine companion that is a joy to share your life with, you will want to carefully read through all the coming Chapters, while always keeping in mind, not just what makes you and your family happy, but what makes your dog happy as well.

Chapter 3: Overview of the Happy Dachshund

"If I could be half the person my dog is,
I'd be twice the human I am."
— Charles Yu

I cannot stress enough how important it is that you understand the basics of any breed, such as size, energy level, intelligence, temperament, and exercise requirements, so that you can truly understand if you are the right person or family for sharing your life with a particular dog.

In the case of the loyal and playful Dachshund, this means gaining some basic knowledge of the history of this small member of the Hound canine category.

Learning about the temperament, health and where this dog's ancestors originally came from will help you choose wisely to ensure that your lifestyle and daily routine can meet this dog's needs.

History

The modern day Dachshund descended from taller versions of German hunting hounds, such as the *"Schweisshund"* and the *"Bibarhund"*, as early as the 17th Century.

Through selective breeding over the period of perhaps 100 years, the legs of these dogs were shortened to make it easier for them to enter badger dens. They have powerful front legs and strong claws for digging and often hunted in packs, chasing a badger out of a den and cornering it until the hunter could arrive.

As is the case with many breeds, the original German Dachshund averaged between 30 and 40 pounds (13 and 18 kilograms), which is considerably larger than the Dachshund of today.

During the 1800's, the Dachshund, that had been developed to excel at hunting both above and below ground, were no longer needed for hunting purposes. They became less and less a hunter and more and more a family pet, which resulted in their standard size being diminished by approximately ten pounds, until the smaller, miniature version was created.

The Dachshund has always been a popular breed and it was only during the great World Wars that their popularity waned because they were associated with Germany. However, it was not long before they regained their popularity and once again were amongst the top ten most popular breeds.

While they have slipped a few places in the last couple of years, the very popular Dachshund has enjoyed being listed amongst the American Kennel Club Top Ten most popular breeds for quite a while. Popularity can be a blessing as well as a curse, because the more popular a small breed becomes, the more likely it will suffer from being bred by unscrupulous puppy mill ventures.

First recognized by the American Kennel Club in 1885 and by the United Kennel Club (UKC) in 1919, the scrappy Dachshund is a small dog with a big dog attitude.

OK, now that you have a basic understanding of the history of the Dachshund, following is the main overview of the breed, which will be the foundation of wisely choosing the right Dachshund and raising a happy and well-behaved dog.

Dachshund Vital Statistics

While every dog is unique, there are standards that are common to each purebred canine, such as height, weight and various coat colors and features. You can also get a pretty good idea of what the puppies will look like when full grown, when you see their parents.

Height and Weight

When measured at the shoulder, the miniature Dachshund stands between 5 and 7 inches (12.7 and 17.7 centimetres) and the standard may stand between 8 and 11 inches (20.3 and 28 centimetres). The miniature Dachshund ideally weighs between 8 and 11 pounds (3.6 and 5 kilograms), while the standard will weigh between 16 and 32 pounds

(7 and 14.5 kilograms). Size will depend on the size of both breed parents, with an average lifespan of between 13 and 15 years, with many living even longer.

Coat Colors and Common Features

This high spirited and independent breed has three distinctively different coat varieties. Perhaps best known as a black and tan smooth coated dog, they can also have a long or wire-haired coat.

The long-haired variety will be slightly wavy, giving the dog an elegant appearance. The wire-haired coat (seen more often in Germany) will be short and thick with a rough outer coat and this dog will have distinctive eyebrows and beard.

Body shape is sturdy with a long back set atop those signature short, strong legs, and all finished off with a tail that gradually tapers to a point.

The Dachshund coat will shed all year round and is usually fairly low maintenance. Some of these dogs will have a single coat and those with a double coat will shed more. Understandably, those with longer coats will require more brushing to keep the coat looking its best while preventing tangles.

Coat colors you can expect to see in a Dachshund are quite varied, including the most common black and tan coat, and many different coat colors or combinations, including black, chocolate, cream, dark brown, fawn, gray (blue), red, tan, wild boar (more often on wire-haired coats), piebald, dappled or tiger-striped brindle.

This dog has medium-length, floppy ears and medium-sized almond-shaped eyes that are usually a darker color. Some dogs that have dappled colored coats may have eyes of two different colors.

How Smart is the Dachshund?

While every dog is surprisingly different even within the same breed, despite what some "experts" might have to say about it, you need to keep in mind that there are *"people smarts"* and *"dog smarts"* and that these two ways of rating intelligence are often widely divergent or in conflict with one another.

If you really want to rate your Dachshund's intelligence, based on what we humans think is *"smart"*, there is a book *("The Intelligence of Dogs")* written in 1994 by Stanley Coren, which has become the standard for rating the particular intelligence of different canine breeds.

While I can agree, in part, with some of the information contained in this book, I can also disagree. I have much personal experience with many breeds, and have found that some dogs that are rated very low on the intelligence scale are also very smart in their own way.

Therefore, I caution you not to pre-handicap your dog's level of intelligence just because of something you may have read in a well-respected book, because each dog has their own unique set of talents and much of how they develop mentally is up to their guardian.

Coren judges canine intelligence of particular purebred canines based on three categories, as follows:

*"**Instinctive Intelligence** – a dog's ability to carry out tasks it was bred to perform, such as guarding, herding, hunting, pointing, retrieving or supplying companionship."*

*"**Adaptive Intelligence** – how well a dog is able to solve problems on its own."*

*"**Working/Obedience Intelligence** – how quickly a dog is able to learn from humans."*

Even though the Dachshund can be a bright little companion, they can have a stubborn streak, a strong prey drive and a mind of their own. Coren places this little hound in the *"Average Working/Obedience Intelligence"* category, likely because they can often have a stubborn or wilful streak.

Please keep in mind that there are always exceptions to every study and a particular breed's degree of intelligence is often related to their early upbringing and how they are trained.

I have had considerable personal experience with this breed, and can tell you that they are fun-loving and usually eager to learn when you use consistent, fair and positive training methods. Yes, they can have a bit of a stubborn streak, and they will not respond well to harsh training, which means that you will have to be patient and find just the right tone when working with this dog.

There is no doubt that with the proper training method and plenty of calm consistency, the Dachshund is easily trainable, and they will be happy and mentally fit so long as they are permitted to spend most of their time in the company of their human guardian.

Temperament of the Dachshund

The Dachshund is a proud and feisty little dog with strong hunting and prey drive instincts that fears nothing. They will chase anything that moves and if you do not have them firmly under your control, they will be out of sight in mere seconds.

While they make wonderful house companions, they need a strong leader to keep them under control, teach them firm rules and boundaries and take them outside for daily "on leash" walks to keep them fit and healthy.

The Dachshund is a dog that requires plenty of companionship and if they don't receive it, and are expected to spend many hours alone, they may become excessive barkers that will not endear you to your neighbor**s.**

As well, the Dachshund is often possessive of toys and food and can display surprising jealousy if you have other pets or children in the home that receive your affection. It will be important to teach this dog their position in the family hierarchy early on, and to immediately put a stop to any signs of jealousy or possessiveness as otherwise, left unchecked, this can lead to unwanted aggressive behavior.

 Every dog needs the discipline of being regularly walked on leash outside of the home each day, as well as the opportunity for off-leash time to run and play fetch or enjoy socializing with other dogs.

 Although the temperament of a Dachshund (or any dog) will vary from dog to dog, and be somewhat dependent upon their first weeks with the breeder, as well as the human guardian who has trained and socialized them during the first few months of their life, generally speaking, this breed displays a loyal and affectionate personality with an alert, temperament.

Proper socializing and teaching basic commands should begin at a young age for the smart Dachshund, who can begin to learn basic commands at ten weeks of age.

This little charmer will generally be an eager to please quick learner that loves to perform and learn new things, so long as you teach with fun and kindness and provide him or her with plenty of praise and tasty treats as rewards for a job well done.

Always keep in mind that any dog, including the Dachshund, can become snappish if teased, provoked or feeling that it must protect itself. Therefore, a guardian should always be watchful when their dog is in the presence of younger children or feeling nervous around much larger dogs.

Most Dachshunds are sturdy, yet loving companions that are great for children that understand how to respect a dog. Remember that this dog has a strong urge to chase and hunt rodents and other small animals. This dog may have a high prey drive, and even when well trained, given the opportunity, they may take off after an interesting scent, such as rabbits, squirrels, other rodents or the neighbor's unsuspecting cat.

Keep in mind that often even with the best training and socialization, a puppy that has inherited "nasty temperament" genes from the breeding parents may still display this tendency. If you have not chosen a reputable breeder, when around other people and animals, you may find yourself apologizing for bad behavior and endlessly making excuses for your otherwise sweet little Dachshund.

 This little character will be just as happy going for a walk with you as they will be learning tricks, going on a road trip, sitting quietly beside you (or on your lap), or snuggled under a blanket while you watch a movie.

The Dachshund will be a loving family dog that is affectionate and totally devoted to the family and while they may not be a particularly good guard dog because of their smaller size, they are fearless and will

give it their best try. This dog will be a superior watchdog that will alert you when anyone is approaching. In fact, if not taught at an early age to stop barking on command, they may bark excessively.

Whatever you teach this dog, at a minimum, make sure that you always get them outside for several, daily, 20-30 minute walks and allow them some off-leash time to run and sniff or play with other smaller dogs.

The Dachshund will be a good choice for active families with older children. While usually good with children and other family pets that have grown up with, very small children may not be the best choice for this dog that will not readily share their toys or tolerate being teased. Small children should be kept away during feeding time.

TIP *The Dachshund prefers their own kind and will usually be suspicious of both unknown dogs and humans. When not trained to live a calm life, they can suffer from attachment issues and loneliness will usually lead to excessive, loud barking that can make you and your neighbors crazy.*

When they are puppies, it's important to engage them in thinking and working activities because they need this stimulation as part of their on-going healthy development.

Just keep in mind that how active you are will likely have a sizeable impact on the health of your Dachshund who will need to eliminate pent up energy by exercising their minds and their bodies so that they can remain a healthy weight.

All puppies are energetic, including the Dachshund puppy, and if you are active with them at a young age, and engage them in training and activities that stretch their minds and bodies, chances are that they will continue to be active into their adult years. On the other hand, if you are an inactive human, the chances are high that your dog will become lazy and overweight, which can shorten their life.

BOTTOM LINE: With this breed is that while the Dachshund will not hesitate to defend his or herself if pushed too far, this is not a trait that you want to encourage, unless you want to spend your days living with an unstable companion.

This is a dog that will be happiest spending all of his or her day being your constant shadow. Depending on the activity level of their human guardian, they will be playful and energetic or less active, often enjoying spending time snoozing next to you or curled up under a warm blanket.

Special Needs

No longer a hunting hound, the Dachshund exists to provide companionship and all the comforts that an indoor lifestyle provides. In other words, this is not a dog to be left alone in a back yard. They are simply not designed to withstand extremes of temperature or being left alone.

FACT *The Dachshund loves to dig, and when you combine their fearless nature with their tenacious tunneling ability and determination, this makes them a talented escape artist.*

Although due to their short legs, they may not be able to leap over a fence, they will certainly use their strong legs to climb fences, dig under fences or find cracks they can squeeze through if they want to get out, and they usually will want to get out because they always want to be where the action is.

This dog is genetically predisposed to a condition called Intervertebral Disc Disease (IVDD). The longer spine means that you must always be careful to support their back when picking them up, and not let them jump from high heights.

These small hounds are also prone to obesity, so don't overfeed and keep food they might get into locked away. Being overweight can exacerbate IVDD.

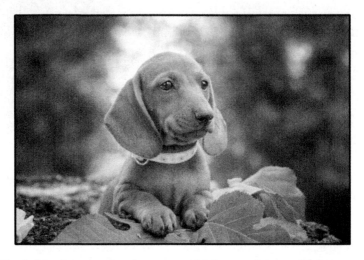

The Dachshund most often has a very high prey drive, which means they cannot be trusted off leash in areas where they could get themselves into trouble.

Remember, fast movement attracts this dog that was bred for hunting mice, rats, rabbits, badgers, random wildlife and other small creatures (such as the neighbor's cat). Killing anything that squeaks is part of their nature so if you want to discourage this killing behavior, don't get them squeaky toys to play with.

Also check under blankets before you sit down because this dog loves to burrow under for a nap.

Even though the Dachshund has short legs, they were bred to be active hunting hounds, which means they are surprisingly energetic. For instance, this companion is easily capable of keeping up on a 10-mile hike. Don't underestimate their exercise needs and capabilities.

Dachshunds are stubborn, tenacious, smart and most are strong willed, and <u>really</u> don't like the rain or the cold.

This can be a frustrating problem if you live in this type of climate and want to housebreak this puppy. In this case, I would strongly recommend the following:

- ❧ provide this puppy with a covered bathroom area;

- ❧ install a doggy door (if you have a back yard), so that he or she can easily and quickly get outside when they feel the urge to go;

- ❧ consider a warm raincoat for this companion.

Finally, never permit this feisty little character to take matters into their own paws by loudly sounding off at other, larger dogs. Permitting this type of behavior is no laughing matter. Don't be another one of those ignorant humans who think it's funny to see a small dog screaming threats at much larger dogs.

To allow this type of behavior is not just highly irresponsible, it's stressful and psychologically unhealthy for your dog. It also contributes to the breed's negative reputation as a nasty yapper, and ultimately can be the cause of an unsafe and disastrous outcome that could be fatal for your beloved companion.

Happy Dachshund Secrets

- ❧ The Dachshund is nicknamed the "Doxy", "Wiener Dog", "Sausage Dog" and "Dash it Hound" and depending on the country, is known by several other names, such as "German Badger Dog", "Perro Saichicha" and "Bassoto". Among hunters they are known as the "Teckel".

- ❧ When literally translated, the word "Dachshund" is German for "badger dog".

- ❧ The Dachshund is often amusingly referred to as being "half a dog high" and "two dogs long".

- ❧ A Dachshund was originally cast as "Toto" in the beloved 1939 Wizard of Oz movie, but as there was strong anti-German sentiment during this time, it was decided that a Cairn terrier should instead be cast in the role.

In a Nutshell

Familiarizing yourself with the Dachshund's size, weight, special needs, and early history, plus understanding their intelligence level, temperament and exercise requirements will help you to decide if the Dachshund is the right dog for you and your family.

Obtaining a comprehensive understanding of the breed's needs will not only save you and your dog from much future grief, but it will be a pre-requisite for raising a content, well-behaved, and happy dog that you are proud to call your best friend and companion.

Chapter 4: Healthy Dachshund = Happy Dog

"Dogs are not our whole life,
but they make our lives whole."
— Roger Caras

If your Dachshund is not physically healthy, he or she will not be a happy canine companion for very long, because suffering from health-related issues can easily create a miserable and ill-mannered dog.

It's prudent that you take the many steps outlined here to help ensure that you are doing all that you can to keep on top of your Dachshund's good health.

Make sure you take the time to choose a veterinarian that can provide yearly check-ups, have your dog spayed or neutered in a timely fashion, choose a healthy diet for him or her, and carefully read this section so that you educate yourself about issues that may adversely affect your dog's health.

As well, take the time to learn a little canine CPR, because doing so may save the life of your own dog, or someone else's.

Below you will find more information on each one of these steps you need to take to raise a healthy and happy Dachshund.

Choose your veterinarian wisely

Some clinics specialize in caring for smaller pets, while some specialize in larger animal care, and others have a wide-ranging area of expertise and will care for all animals, including livestock and reptiles.

Choosing a good veterinary clinic will be very similar to choosing the right health care clinic or doctor for your own personal health, because you want to ensure that your puppy or adult dog receives the quality care they deserve. A good place to begin your search will be by asking other dog owners where they take their furry friends and whether they are happy with the service they receive.

 It's also a good idea to take your Dachshund into your chosen clinic several times before they actually need to be there for any treatment, so that they are not fearful of the new smells and unfamiliar surroundings.

Consider timely neutering or spaying

There are varying opinions on the topic of the best time to neuter or spay your young Dachshund. One thing that most veterinarians do agree on is that earlier spaying or neutering, between 4 and 6 months of age, can be a better choice than waiting longer.

Keep in mind that non-neutered or spayed males and females are more likely to display aggression related to sexual behaviour, than are dogs that have been neutered or spayed.

For instance, fighting, particularly in male dogs that is directed at other males, is less common after neutering. The intensity of other types of aggression, such as irritable aggression in females will be totally eliminated by spaying, so make that appointment at the vet's office and get it done.

Effects on General Temperament: many dog owners often become needlessly worried that a neutered or spayed dog will lose their vigor, when in fact, many unwanted, aggressive qualities, resulting from hormonal impact, may resolve after surgery, and you will be acting as a conscientious, informed, and caring guardian.

Effects on Escape and Roaming: a neutered or spayed Dachshund is less likely to wander, and castrated male dogs have the tendency to patrol smaller sized outdoor areas and are less likely to participate in territorial conflicts with perceived opponents.

Possible Weight Gain: while metabolic changes that occur after spaying or neutering can cause some puppies to gain weight, often the real culprit for any weight gain is the human who feels guilty for subjecting their puppy to this medical procedure, and in an attempt to make themselves feel better, they feed more treats or meals to their companion.

 If you notice weight gain after neutering or spaying your Dachshund puppy, simply adjust their food and treat consumption as needed and once stitches are healed, make sure that they are receiving adequate daily exercise.

<u>Educate yourself with respect to vaccination</u>

 It has now become common practice to vaccinate adult dogs every three years, and if your veterinarian is insisting on a yearly vaccination for your puppy, you need to ask them why, because to do otherwise is considered by many professionals to be *"over vaccinating"*.

Whether or not your dog actually needs a booster can be determined with a simple blood test at your vet's office, so be proactive, and ask for a blood test.

Puppies need to be vaccinated in order to provide them with protection against four common and serious diseases referred to as *"DAPP"*, which stands for Distemper, Adenovirus, Parainfluenza and Parvo Virus.

Approximately one week after your puppy has completed all three sets of primary DAPP vaccinations, they will be fully protected from those specific diseases.

Be aware of the health conditions that may affect your dog

While a healthy, happy Dachshund may live to be 12 to 14 years (more or less), and with proper care they may not suffer from any of the below noted health concerns, it is prudent to list all concerns possibly associated with this breed so that you have a clear understanding of problems that *"may"* affect your dog, including:

Accidental Injury: more than disease or illness, the Dachshund is more likely to suffer from back and neck disc injury as a result of their very short legs and elongated back. For instance, this dog can easily injure his or herself by jumping from a chair or couch. A well-meaning human can also cause back injury if they do not properly support this dog's long back when they are picked up.

Small dogs with fearless attitudes and strong prey drive, such as the Dachshund, should always be kept on leash because they may place themselves into all sorts of circumstances whereby they could easily be injured when they are not under your complete control.

Also, small dogs are NOT usually suitable pets for young children, who may accidentally hurt them or drop them. Children are usually loud, fast moving, boisterous and oftentimes clumsy, which is a combination for danger around a small dog that might suffer all manner of injuries at the hands of a young child that meant well.

Further, most dogs will feel overwhelmed by the loud, shrill voices and quick movements that young children can't help making with the result being that the dog may experience stress, fear and even defensive biting while it tries to defend itself from what it may believe to be a threat or an invasion of their personal space.

Luxating Patella (see picture): the Dachshund breed has the 8ᵗʰ worse case of this health problem. This slipping kneecap condition is a common defect seen in many breeds that may also be caused by accidentally falling or jumping from a height. Often you will see a dog with this problem appear to be skipping down the road as they occasionally lift one leg when the kneecap slips out of the patellar groove and the leg locks up. Surgery is the treatment option for this condition, although many dogs live a relatively normal life with this defect.

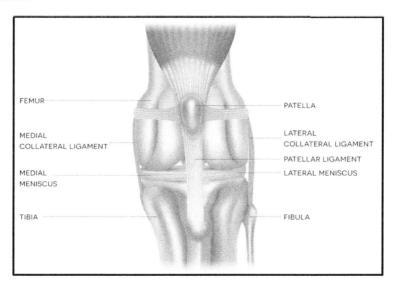

Hip & Elbow Dysplasia (pictured for hip): is a degenerative disease in which the hip or elbow joint becomes weakened due to abnormal growth. Depending upon the severity of the disease, treatment will involve medication or surgery. Screening of the parents cannot guarantee that puppies will not be born with this problem.

Dysplasia occurs when the bone slips out of its rightful place in the hip or elbow socket. When the bone is out of joint, it can cause the dog to limp or it might cause total limb lameness. Over time, the wear and tear on the joints can lead to painful inflammation, which may necessitate a surgical repair. In more mild cases, other treatment options include pain medications and anti-inflammatories.

Factors that have an influence include nutrition, a dog's weight, a dog's environment and the condition of the hips of its parents.

Intervertebral Disc Disease (IVDD): as a result of this dog's body generally significantly longer than they are tall, they are at the highest risk of suffering from these back and neck problems.

The intervertebral disks function to cushion the spine, and if they bulge or rupture, can cause nerve problems as well as loss of coordination and severe pain. If this problem is not treated, it can result in permanent weakness or paralysis. One out of every four Dachshunds will suffer from a disc problem during their lifetime.

Legg-Calve Perthes: this is a more serious, but less common, disease of the hip joint involving degeneration of the head of the femur, which causes severe pain and lameness.

Progressive Retinal Atrophy (PRA): causes degeneration of the retina, which is part of the eye. The retina is the part that senses visual information and sends it to the brain. Degeneration of this vital part of the eye eventually will lead to blindness. This disease usually appears between 3 and 5 years of age. A simple DNA test is available to determine (without waiting for symptoms to appear).

Cataracts (see picture): the Dachshund can suffer from cataracts that cause the lens of the eye to become opaque or cloudy, leading to blindness.

While this disease usually occurs in old age, it can also appear in a younger dog and treatment involves surgical removal.

Technically speaking, a cataract is an opacity that forms in the lens of the eye and it can partially or completely obstruct your dog's vision. Though cataracts are not painful, there is a slight risk that the cataract could slip out of place and float around the eye or it could become stuck in the tear duct, blocking fluid drainage.

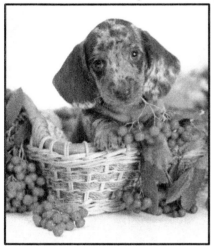

Unfortunately, cataracts cannot be prevented, especially if it is a condition your puppy inherited genetically. If the cataract is caught while still in the early stages, however, your vet may be able to take steps to slow the progression and maybe even save your dog's vision. In some cases, a dog's vision can be restored by surgically removing the cataract, however, there is a fairly long recovery period for this kind of surgery.

Glaucoma: this eye disease, which is usually caused by an increase of fluid pressure in the eye, can cause permanent damage to the dog's vision in the affected eye or eyes, which can lead to blindness.

Persistent Pupillary Membrane: this inherited disease is caused when remnants of fetal membrane, which is a source of blood supply for the fetus, continues to persist after birth of the puppy. Under normal circumstances this membrane atrophies between birth and 4 to 8 weeks, but when the atrophy is not complete, strands of the membrane connect to the lens of the eye, which can then cause cataracts.

Corneal Dystrophy: this disease is a change in the eye usually attributed to aging, causing fluid leakage that appears as a bluish color in the inner layer of the cornea.

Dry Eye: also called *"dry eye syndrome"* or *"Keratoconjunctivitis"*, is a loss of tear film over the surface of the dog's eyes which causes drying and inflammation of the cornea of the dog's eye. Dogs suffering from dry eye will blink more often and the tissues lining the eyelids may become swollen. Unless the condition is severe (with discharge from the eye), treatment will involve applying artificial tear medication and possibly an antibiotic ointment to counteract any bacterial infection.

Inherited Deafness: this can occur in dogs with dappled colored coats. In most breeds this is associated with white coat coloration as this is linked to the piebald and/or merle genes. Deafness usually occurs in puppies within a few weeks of birth and it can occur in only one ear or both ears. There is no cure and puppies that are deaf in both ears are often euthanized because they are accident-prone or startle easily, which can lead to biting, and can be difficult to train.

Demodectic Mange: is a skin disease known by several names, including *"red mange"*, *"follicular mange"* or *"puppy mange",* caused by the Demodex canis mite, and usually in young dogs or puppies. This is a disease that is caused by a weak, poorly developed or suppressed immune system that is unable to keep the spread of these mites, which are passed from mother to puppy, under control.

Most puppies are immune to the effect of these microscopic mites and the few that are not develop hair loss, or red, crusty lesions, usually around the head. Most will heal without intervention as the puppy matures and the dog's immune system grows stronger. In persistent cases, treatment involves the application of topical medication applied to the skin.

Follicular Dysplasia: is a genetic condition that causes hair loss due to structural abnormality or weakened hair follicles, which can also be caused by injury or excessive grooming. There is no cure and this more commonly occurs on the back of the dog, near the tail.

Color Dilution Alopecia (CDA): known also as color mutant alopecia, blue balding or blue Doberman syndrome, is a type of hair loss affecting only the colored areas of hair on dogs that have dilute colored (blue, blue fawn, fawn) coats. Hair loss usually begins in the middle of the dog's back and can spread to include the rest of the body. There is no treatment and thankfully for the affected dog, there is no accompanying itching.

Pattern Baldness: is a harmless skin condition causing a gradual thinning or complete loss of hair around the dog's temples and ears, underneath the neck and abdomen, and on the backs of the thighs. It does not cause itching and the dog's skin and coat appear otherwise normal. There is no treatment for this cosmetic condition other than ensuring a good food source and adding skin and coat supplements to the diet.

Pyoderma: is a bacterial infection of the dog's skin that causes itching and redness that can lead to lesions on the skin that are similar to pimples. Treatment involves shampoo and antibiotic creams.

Acanthosis Nigricans: this less common skin condition, that does not affect the dog's health, causes the skin to darken, thicken and lose the hair. This usually begins in the dog's armpits and then progresses to the groin and stomach areas.

Von Willebrand's Disease: is a blood disorder similar to hemophilia in humans where blood does not clot properly, which means that if the dog becomes injured, they are more likely to suffer from excessive bleeding episodes. There is a simple DNA test available to rule out this disease at any time, rather than waiting for symptoms to appear. To ensure that the puppy you may be considering is as healthy as possible, always ask questions about whether the parents of a particular puppy have been screened and are free from the types of health problems that may be inherent in the breed.

Epilepsy: is considered a neurological problem. While the most common cause of seizures is idiopathic epilepsy, which is an inherited form of epilepsy, many factors can cause seizures, including physical trauma, such as a head injury, and it is very important to have a dog diagnosed if seizures begin.

Cushing's Disease: there are three forms of Cushing's Disease and most dogs suffer from the more common form, *"Pituitary Dependent PD"*, which is a slow growing form of cancer that is located in the pituitary gland caused by an increase in cortisone as a result of a benign tumor. There are many symptoms including obesity, increased thirst and urination, loss of hair, bruising, lack of energy, and excessive panting. Once diagnosed, symptoms will be treated with daily oral medication.

Hypothyroidism: is a condition resulting from an inadequate production of thyroid hormone and is treated with medication. Symptoms can include weight gain or obesity, constant hunger, reduced energy and a coarser feel to the dog's coat texture. Blood samples will be taken in order to test for a malfunctioning thyroid.

Diabetes: is one of the most common canine hormonal diseases that can occur at quite an early age (18-months) but may not be diagnosed until much later in the dog's life, between 7 and 10 years of age. Interestingly, 70% of diabetes is seen in female dogs. Usually, the first sign of this disease is a normal appetite, with an increased consumption of water and weight loss. Also, the sudden onset of cataracts may indicate an underlying diabetes cause.

Urinary Stones (Urolithiasis): is a urinary problem where crystals or stones form in the dog's urinary tract or the kidney, urethra or bladder, which then blocks the flow of urine. Symptoms involve pain and blood in the dog's urine and a dog suffering from this problem may start to urinate in unusual places, behave depressed and lose their appetite. Treatment may involve diet changes or medication, and in severe cases, surgery.

Mitral Valve Disease (MVD): is a degeneration of the mitral heart valve that can lead to heart failure. If a dog has this problem, the blood will flow back into the chamber, which can cause the chamber to enlarge, which then can cause other problems, including an irregular heartbeat, constricted windpipe, or flowing back into the lungs.

The first sign of mitral valve disease is a heart murmur, which can usually only be heard with a stethoscope. Symptoms include fainting, coughing, increased blood pressure, tiredness and reluctance to exercise. There is no cure and beyond replacing the valve, management involves various drug therapies to improve the dog's quality of life.

Sebaceous Gland Tumors: are benign cysts or a sac filled with fluid or semi-solid material. If they become walled off from the dog's body, they may feel like a little pea underneath the skin.

These harmless cysts are usually caused by a build-up of oil or a blocked oil gland in the dog's skin, and when left alone, they will usually resolve themselves. Unless they are somehow interfering with the dog's health, it is recommended to leave them alone rather than attempting to squeeze them, which can lead to infection.

Bloat (Emergency Gastrointestinal Syndrome): is a life-threatening, common occurrence that can affect any deep-chested canine, and 50% of dogs that develop bloat do not survive. This condition can happen very quickly, especially if you feed your dog right after vigorous exercise, or if they are a very fast eater and gulp in large quantities of air with their food.

The stomach then distends with gas and fluid which can cause the stomach to twist 180-degrees or more. When the stomach is closed off, the food is then trapped inside where it will ferment and cause the stomach to bulge. The bulging stomach can then interfere with blood circulation and obstruct veins in the abdomen, which creates low blood pressure, followed by shock and damage to internal organs.

Bloat is a serious, life-threatening condition that requires immediate veterinary intervention. If you have a deep chested dog that tends to gulp their food, get them a slow feeder type of bowl to slow down their eating process and never feed them immediately after exercise or having had a large drink of water.

When you take good care of your happy Dachshund's health, and they come from a trusted breeder, he or she may never have to suffer from any of the above-noted list of health problems.

Educate Yourself About Common Canine Diseases and Viruses

While your dog may never suffer from a common disease or virus, in order to ensure the safety and health of your happy Dachshund, you need to be aware of the many common diseases and viruses that could detrimentally affect the health of your dog.

Always watch out for the symptoms of the following common diseases and if you suspect that your dog has been infected, contact your vet immediately.

Distemper (sometimes called *"hard pad disease"*): is a contagious, serious, and deadly viral illness that is spread through the air or by direct or indirect contact with a dog (or other animal) that is already infected (such as ferrets, raccoons, foxes, skunks and wolves), that can also cause thickening of the pads on the feet or nose.

Early symptoms include fever, loss of appetite and mild eye inflammation that may only last a day or two, with symptoms becoming more serious and noticeable as the disease progresses. There is no known cure.

Adenovirus: causes infectious canine hepatitis, which can range in severity from very mild to very serious. The treatment focuses on management of symptoms, and the condition can sometimes result in death. Symptoms can vary and may include coughing, loss of appetite, increased thirst and urination, tiredness, vomiting and seizures.

Canine Parainfluenza Virus (CPIV): also referred to as *"canine influenza virus"*, *"greyhound disease"* or *"race flu"*, which is easily spread through the air or by coming into contact with respiratory secretions.
While it is usually a self-limiting virus that will run its course within a couple of weeks, in severe cases and without antibiotic treatment, it may be fatal.

Symptoms can include a dry, hacking cough, difficulty breathing, wheezing, runny nose and eyes, sneezing, fever, loss of appetite, tiredness, depression and possible pneumonia. In cases where only a cough exists, tests will be required to determine whether the cause of the cough is the parainfluenza virus or the less serious *"kennel cough"*.

Canine Parvovirus (CPV): is a highly contagious viral illness affecting puppies and dogs, foxes, coyotes and wolves. Symptoms include vomiting, bloody diarrhoea, weight loss, and lack of appetite. Without prompt and proper treatment, dogs that have severe parvovirus infections can die within 48 to 72 hours.

Treatment will involve addressing dehydration and correcting electrolyte imbalances by administering intravenous fluids. Anti-inflammatory and antibiotic drugs are also given to control or prevent septicaemia, as well as drugs to control diarrhoea and vomiting.

Other Diseases and Viruses to Be Aware Of

What is Zoonotic? Zoonotic means a contagious disease that can be spread between both animals and humans.

Rabies: is a viral, zoonotic disease transmitted by coming into contact with the saliva of an infected animal, usually through a bite. The virus travels to the brain along the nerves and once symptoms develop (usually marked by a change in temperament), after a prolonged period of suffering, death is almost certainly inevitable. There is no treatment.

In most countries, vaccination against rabies is mandatory between the ages of twelve and sixteen weeks. If you plan to travel out of State or across country borders, you will need to make sure that your dog has an up-to-date Rabies Vaccination Certificate (NASPHV form 51) indicating they have been inoculated against rabies.

Leishmaniasis: is a contagious zoonotic infection caused by a parasite and is transmitted by a bite from a sand fly. While treatment involves the administration of a special drug (sodium stibogluconate), there is no definitive answer for effectively combating Leishmaniasis (especially since one vaccine will not prevent the known multiple species), with the prognosis often being fatal.

Symptoms include loss of appetite, diarrhoea, severe weight loss, exercise intolerance, vomiting, nosebleed, tarry feces, fever, pain in the joints, excessive thirst and urination, inflammation of the muscles, and death from kidney failure.

Lyme Disease: is one of the most common zoonotic tick-borne diseases in the world, which is transmitted by Borrelia bacteria found in the deer or sheep tick. Symptoms of this disease in a young or adult dog include recurrent lameness from joint inflammation, loss of appetite, depression, stiff walk with arched back, sensitivity to touch, swollen

lymph nodes, fever, kidney damage, as well as rare heart or nervous system complications.

Control of the symptoms involves a lengthy course of antibiotic treatment in order to completely eliminate the organism.

Rocky Mountain Spotted Fever (RMSF): is a zoonotic disease transmitted by both the American dog tick and the RMSF tick, which must be attached to the dog for a minimum of five hours in order to transmit the disease.

Common symptoms include fever, reduced appetite, depression, painful joints, lameness, vomiting and diarrhoea, and some dogs may develop heart abnormalities, pneumonia, kidney failure, liver damage, or even neurological signs, such as seizures or unsteady, wobbly or stumbling gait. Treatment involves a 2-3 week course of antibiotics (Doxycycline or Tetracycline).

Ehrlichiosis: a tick-borne disease transmitted by both the brown dog tick and the Lone Star Tick, with common symptoms including depression, reduced appetite, fever, stiff and painful joints and bruising. The signs of infection typically occur less than a month after a tick bite and last for approximately four weeks. There is no vaccine available. Treatment involves a long course of antibiotics.

Anaplasmosis: deer ticks (**pictured**) and Western blacklegged ticks are carriers of the bacteria that transmit canine Anaplasmosis. However, there is also another form of Anaplasmosis (caused by a different bacteria) that is carried by the brown dog tick.

Because the deer tick also carries other diseases, some animals may be at risk of developing more than one tick-borne disease at the same time. Signs are similar to Ehrlichiosis and include painful joints, diarrhoea, fever, and vomiting, as well as possible nervous system disorders. Treatment involves administering the antibiotic Doxycycline for a 30-day period.

Tick Paralysis (pictured): this zoonotic infection is caused when ticks attach themselves to the skin and secrete a neurotoxin that affects the nervous system. Affected dogs show signs of weakness and limpness approximately one week after being first bitten.

Symptoms usually begin with a change in pitch of the dog's usual bark, and weakness in the rear legs that eventually involves all four legs, followed by the dog showing difficulty breathing and swallowing. Your dog can die if not diagnosed and properly treated by removal of the tick.

Canine Coronavirus: this highly contagious intestinal disease, which is spread through the feces of contaminated dogs, while now found worldwide, can be destroyed by most commonly available disinfectants. Symptoms include diarrhoea, vomiting and weight loss or anorexia. There is a vaccine available, which is usually given to puppies, because they are more susceptible at a young age. This vaccine is also given to show dogs that have a higher risk of exposure to the disease.

Leptospirosis: is a worldwide zoonotic bacterial infection that can affect humans and many different kinds of animals, including dogs. If left untreated, there is potential for both dogs and humans to die from this disease.

The good news is that this virus is usually treated with antibiotics and supportive care, and because you can protect your dog with a vaccination, it makes sense to vaccinate against this disease if you and your dog live in an area considered a hot spot for leptospirosis.

Be aware that allergies can adversely affect your dog's health

You may be surprised to learn that dogs can suffer from allergies in much the same way that people can. Not only can the Dachshund develop allergies to certain food ingredients, but he can also develop inhalant or contact allergies. The general signs of allergies include the following:

- Itchy red skin (**see picture below**)
- Itchy or runny eyes
- Licking the base of the tail
- Sneezing or coughing
- Ear infections
- Diarrhea
- Snoring from throat inflammation
- Chewing the paws

Some of the things that your dog can be allergic to include grass, weeds, pollen, mold spores, dust, dander, feathers, cigarette smoke, prescription drugs, perfumes, and cleaning products. They can also be allergic to certain flea and tick products, so be very careful which one you choose. You should also never use products on your dog that are not designed specifically for dogs – this includes shampoo.

One of the most common complaints discussed at the veterinarian's office when they see dogs obsessively scratching, biting, licking and chewing at their skin or paws is possible allergies, and there can be many triggers. When you educate yourself, you can help ensure your Dachshund never has to suffer from allergies and can lead a healthier and happier life.

Environmental allergies: what many of us humans seem to forget is that our dogs can develop allergies to dust, chemicals, grass, mould, pollen, car exhaust, various forms of smoke, or flea and tick preparations, as well as allergies to materials such as wool or cotton, and chemicals found in washing soap or chemicals found in cleaning products you use around your home.

Visual symptoms are usually first noticed on the dog's stomach, inside of their legs, and at their tail or paws. Because many allergies are seasonal, our dogs will often be more affected in the spring or fall, with some airborne irritants inhaled by your dog resulting in coughing, sneezing or watery eyes.

Pay attention and if you think that your dog may have come in contact with an irritant found somewhere in your environment, first give them a cleansing bath, with the proper canine shampoo and conditioner.

Junk food allergies: *"True"* food allergies usually account for only about 10% of allergy problems in our canine friends.

Be aware that itching, chewing and chronic ear infections are not actually caused by food allergies, but rather are the result of a suppressed immune system, which is the result of your dog eating a low-quality diet. Food sensitivity issues can often be completely resolved by changing your dog's diet to a high-quality food that is more easily digested.

For instance, check food ingredients because far too many dog food products contain gluten ingredients that are common allergens to our fur friends, such as corn, wheat and soybeans. Become a label reader and ask questions, before you choose your dog's food.

Take the Time to Learn a Little Canine CPR

Of course, nobody wants to find his or herself in a situation where the life of their precious canine companion is put at risk. However, the reality is that accidents happen, and therefore knowing a little bit about how to help save your beloved furry friend is time well spent.

First of all, remember to handle an injured dog very carefully and gently. A dog that is traumatized, fearful or in pain, even one that is usually gentle, may lash out and try to bite.

Consider taking a class, because there are many animal CPR courses being offered these days through community educational systems or even online.

It's also a good idea to put together a canine first aid kit, both at home and in your vehicle, in case of emergencies, that includes the following items:

- 🐾 Antiseptic Wash for wounds (hydrogen peroxide)
- 🐾 Blanket
- 🐾 Gauze Bandaging
- 🐾 Kwik Stop styptic powder
- 🐾 Medical Tape

- 🐾 Nail Clippers
- 🐾 Non-Stick Bandages for wounds
- 🐾 Scissors
- 🐾 Sterile Eye Wash
- 🐾 Tick Twister
- 🐾 Towel
- 🐾 Tweezers
- 🐾 Wash cloth

It would also be prudent to obtain a copy of the American Red Cross emergency techniques called *"Saving Your Pet With CPR"*, and familiarize yourself with the proper way to administer CPR to a dog.

Artificial Respiration Step by Step

If your dog becomes unconscious, depending upon what happened to them, they may stop breathing and if they stop breathing, they will go into cardiac arrest, when the heart stops beating and the dog dies.

However, after breathing stops, and before cardiac arrest, the heart can continue to beat for several minutes and this is when performing cardiopulmonary resuscitation (CPR) or artificial respiration can save your dog's life.

Step 1: place your dog on his or her side on a flat surface.

Step 2: check to make sure that your dog has actually stopped breathing by watching for the rise and fall of their chest and feel for their breath on your hand. Check the color of your dog's gums, because lack of oxygen will make them turn blue.

Step 3: check that the dog's airway is clear and there is nothing stuck in their mouth or throat by extending the head and neck and opening your dog's mouth.

If there is an object blocking their throat, pull the tongue outward and use your fingers or pliers to get a firm grip on the object so that you can pull it free from the dog's throat. If you cannot reach the object that appears to be blocking the dog's airway passage, you will have to use the Heimlich Manoeuver to try and dislodge it (see below).

Step 4: so long as the dog's airway is not blocked, you can lift their chin to straighten out the neck and begin rescue breathing.

Step 5: hold the dog's muzzle and close their mouth, put your mouth over the dog's nose and blow gently – just enough to cause the dog's chest to rise.

Step 6: wait long enough for the air you just breathed into the dog's lungs to leave before giving another breath.

Step 7: continue giving one gentle breath every 3 seconds as long as the heart is still beating and until your dog starts to breathe on their own.

Canine Heimlich Manoeuvre

If breath won't go in, the airway may be blocked. In this case, you will need to turn your dog upside down, with his or her back held against your chest.

Wrap your arms around the dog and clasp your hands together just below the dog's rib cage (since the dog is being held upside down, this will be actually above the rib cage, in the abdomen).

Using both arms, give five sharp thrusts to the abdomen, and then check the dog's mouth or airway for the object. If the object is visible, remove it, and give two more rescue breaths.

CPR Step by Step

If your Dachshund's heart has stopped beating, then CPR must be started immediately and ideal would be to have one person performing the artificial respiration, while the other performs the CPR.

Step 1: put your dog on his or her side on a flat surface.

Step 2: feel for your dog's pulse or heartbeat by placing one hand over his or her left side, just behind the front leg.

Step 3: place the palm of your hand on your dog's rib cage over his or her heart, with your other hand on top of the first (for puppies, put just your thumb on one side of the chest and the rest of your fingers on the other side).

Step 4: press down and release, compressing the dog's chest approximately one inch (2-3 centimetres) and squeeze and release 80 to 100 times every minute.

While it's always the hope that you may never need to, if your dog is not breathing and there is no pulse, knowing what steps to take in an emergency (which includes how to do the doggy Heimlich Manoeuvre or apply compressions), could literally save the life of your own dog or maybe even someone else's.

In a Nutshell

While your dog may never suffer from any of the diseases known to affect this breed, you will want to know what *may* afflict your dog because being aware of the signs can help them live a longer life. As well, familiarizing yourself with emergency CPR procedures in the following American Red Cross chart could help you save your dog's life.

It is also prudent to take the time to choose a veterinarian that can provide yearly check-ups, have your dog spayed or neutered in a timely fashion and educate yourself about required vaccinations.

Taking the steps outlined in this Chapter will help ensure that your Dachshund will always have the best opportunity to be healthy and happy throughout your lifelong journey together.

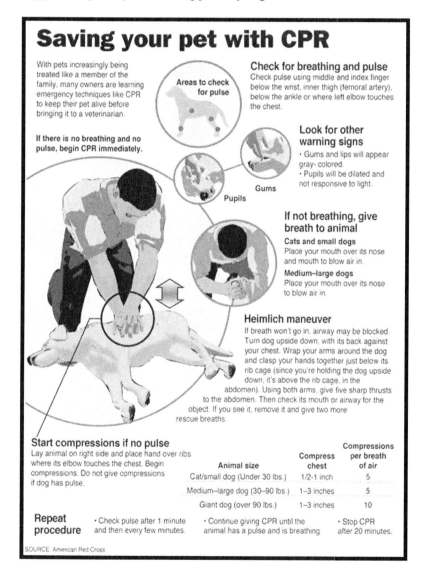

Saving your pet with CPR

With pets increasingly being treated like a member of the family, many owners are learning emergency techniques like CPR to keep their pet alive before bringing it to a veterinarian.

Areas to check for pulse

If there is no breathing and no pulse, begin CPR immediately.

Pupils

Gums

Check for breathing and pulse
Check pulse using middle and index finger below the wrist, inner thigh (femoral artery), below the ankle or where left elbow touches the chest.

Look for other warning signs
· Gums and lips will appear gray- colored.
· Pupils will be dilated and not responsive to light.

If not breathing, give breath to animal

Cats and small dogs
Place your mouth over its nose and mouth to blow air in.

Medium–large dogs
Place your mouth over its nose to blow air in.

Heimlich maneuver
If breath won't go in, airway may be blocked. Turn dog upside down, with its back against your chest. Wrap your arms around the dog and clasp your hands together just below its rib cage (since you're holding the dog upside down, it's above the rib cage, in the abdomen). Using both arms, give five sharp thrusts to the abdomen. Then check its mouth or airway for the object. If you see it, remove it and give two more rescue breaths.

Start compressions if no pulse
Lay animal on right side and place hand over ribs where its elbow touches the chest. Begin compressions. Do not give compressions if dog has pulse.

Animal size	Compress chest	Compressions per breath of air
Cat/small dog (Under 30 lbs.)	1/2-1 inch	5
Medium–large dog (30–90 lbs.)	1–3 inches	5
Giant dog (over 90 lbs.)	1–3 inches	10

Repeat procedure
· Check pulse after 1 minute and then every few minutes.
· Continue giving CPR until the animal has a pulse and is breathing
· Stop CPR after 20 minutes.

SOURCE: American Red Cross

Chapter 5: Let Your Dog BE a Happy Dog

"Don't make the mistake of treating your dogs
like humans, or they'll treat you like dogs."
— Martha Scott

This chapter is written to alert you to the fact that far too many of us humans have the tendency to treat our dogs more like human fur children than dogs.

You need to understand that not allowing your Dachshund to be *"dog-like"* is very important when we're talking about THEIR happiness, because treating a dog like a human can ultimately result in <u>YOU</u> creating any number of behavioral issues.

<u>Your Dachshund is Not a Child</u>

While this might sound like a strange Chapter title, there is no doubt that many humans simply don't allow their dogs to actually BE dogs, because they are too busy confusing their dog by attributing human emotions to them, and treating them like children.

The urge to treat the Dachshund like a delicate child that needs to be dressed up in the latest designer fashions, wear pink tutus and rhinestone collars is especially strong with smaller breeds.

Yes, some dogs, such as the Dachshund, may need to wear clothing to keep warm and dry, and depending on where they live, their guardian may need to provide them with protection from the cold and rain during the winter months. However, if the only reason you are dressing up your dog is because it makes you laugh, or appeals to a frustrated maternal instinct, this is NOT a healthy relationship.

Also keep in mind that if you live in a warm climate, you may want to provide them with a cooling vest during warmer summer months when they are walking outside in the sunshine.

When your Dachshund is a full-grown adult, you will definitely want to begin more complicated or advanced training sessions. They will enjoy it when you have the desire and patience, and they have the willingness.

If you and your Dachshund are really enjoying learning new tricks together, you might want to advance to teaching them the hand signals for *"commando crawl"*, how to *"speak"* or to *"jump through the human hoop"*, and you might want to also consider getting them involved in a fun canine sport, like Agility.

 The only restriction to how far you can go with training your adult Dachshund will be your imagination and their personal energy level, ability or desire to perform.

Every dog has a uniquely wonderful set of gifts to share with their human counterparts, if only us humans would listen. They *"tell"* us when they are unhappy, frightened, bored, nervous, and when they are under-exercised, yet often we do not pay attention, or we just think they are being badly behaved.

Many humans today are deciding to have dogs instead of children and then attempting to manipulate their dogs into being small (or large) furry children. This is having a seriously detrimental effect upon the health, happiness and behavior of our canine companions.

Single, lonely people often have dogs, which is just fine, so long as the human side of the equation doesn't expect their canine counterpart to fulfill what humans require on an emotional level, because this is very confusing to a dog who needs their human to lead them.

In order to be the best guardians for our dogs, we humans must have a better understanding of what our dogs need from us, rather than what we need from them, so that they can live in safety, harmony and security within our human environment.

Sadly, many of us humans are not well equipped to give our dogs what they really need and that is why there are so many homeless, abandoned and frustrated dogs and so many overflowing rescue facilities.

PERSONAL EXPERIENCE: As a professional dog whisperer who is challenged with the task of finding amicable solutions for canine/human relationships that have gone off the rails, I can tell you with certainty that once humans understand what needs to be changed and actually take the steps to do the work required, almost every stressful canine/human relationship can be turned into a happy one.

The sad part is that many humans are simply not willing or able to really understand the breed they are choosing, or willing or able to do the consistent work and devote the time necessary to ensuring that their chosen dog's needs are truly met.

Almost ALL canine problems, both mentally and physically, are a direct result of ignorance, time restraints or unwillingness on the part of the human guardian to choose the right dog and then learn what their dog truly needs.

First and foremost, our dogs need to be respected for their unique canine qualities.

For millennia, dog has been considered *"Man's best friend"*. In today's society, when we want to do the best for our canine companions and create a harmonious relationship, we humans need to spend more time receiving the proper training WE need, so that we can learn how we humans can be dog's best friend.

Any dog can be your *"best friend"* providing that YOU educate yourself and put in the work. This is a universal truth that applies to any canine breed, including the toy-sized Dachshund.

If you are considering this energetic and fearless small hound for your family, be certain that you can involve them in routines and tasks that will engage both their body and their mind, because doing so will ensure that you are raising a happy dog that never has to suffer from behavioral issues or poor health.

In a Nutshell

It's important to understand that no matter the size of your chosen canine friend, you actually need to let your dog BE a dog if you want to raise a happy and healthy companion.

While being overly protective, carrying this small dog everywhere and treating them like a fur covered child may be something YOU need, it's not what THEY need, and can create much confusion that often will lead to behavioral issues sooner or later in life.

Chapter 6: Every Happy Dachshund Wants Exercise

"The dog lives for the day,
the hour, even the moment."
— Robert Scott

This breed will usually require a moderate daily physical exercise regimen, that also includes going out for 2-3 on-leash walks, walking properly at your side every day, because this will result in a strong bond of trust and respect between you and your dog that translates to both a healthy body and a healthy mind.

If you cannot commit to the time required to ensure your dog receives regular exercise each day, that engages both mind and body, this will soon be a very unhealthy, overweight, unhappy dog that could develop multiple health and behavior issues.

Minimum Daily Exercise Requirements

You will need to get your dog outside every day for a minimum of two or three 20 to 30 minute, on-leash, disciplined walks where they are walking at your side without pulling, and paying close attention to your commands.

Once properly leash trained and heeding basic commands, the Dachshund will also enjoy the reward of some off-leash freedom at a securely fenced local dog park where they can run, socialize, play with other similar-sized dogs or perhaps chase a ball or small Frisbee.

 *T**he intelligent Dachshund will usually enjoy participating in Agility, Conformation, Earth Dog trials, Field trials, Flyball, Rally, Racing, Tracking, Barn Hunt, Obedience, Trick Training, and more.***

Depending on your training, this proud and feisty little companion may be friendly with strangers, he or she may be reserved or suspicious of those they don't know, or some may display non-stop barking toward any animal or person getting too close for their comfort. If your puppy begins to display this sort of unsettling behavior, you must immediately curtail this type of outburst and firmly teach him or her that this is NOT acceptable behavior.

To do nothing about it sends an unspoken message to your dog that you approve of this type of crazed behavior and you will have contributed toward creating a noisy, loud barking scene that could be very difficult to correct.

Always be proactive and teach your dog what is, and what is not acceptable. When you draw a firm line in the sand and consistently enforce rules and boundaries, you will have given your loyal and loving little Dachshund the best opportunity for a happy and stress-free life.

Your dog needs to learn how to properly greet other dogs and humans, and part of making this a stress-free situation is letting your dog know that YOU will keep them safe. Otherwise, they may live a life of nervous anxiety, feeling they must always be on the alert to defend their space.

Keeping your Dachshund "safe" does not mean always picking them up when an unknown dog approaches. Many humans get into this bad habit. Don't let this be you, because you will be teaching your dog that all other dogs are not to be trusted and this will inevitably lead to creating a nervous, fearful and unstable companion. If you are uncertain about another dog approaching, simply place yourself between your dog and the approaching dog until you are certain a friendly greeting will be the outcome.

Keep in mind that the miniature version of this small companion will usually be curious, fun loving and playful, and because they are a smaller size, they are easy to travel with.

TIP: get the miniature Dachshund used to quietly travelling inside a handy *"Sherpa"* bag when he or she is a small puppy. When you take the time to do this, this little companion will easily travel anywhere with you, even on the local bus service or as carry-on luggage on a plane.

<u>Ideal Daily Exercise Requirements</u>

A fully-grown Dachshund can be a curious, energetic and playful dog or (depending on you) more of a lazy couch potato. However, both will need mental and physical stimulation from disciplined walks and daily exercise, and that may include trick training or canine sports in order to maintain a happy disposition and a healthy weight.

Keep in mind that, depending on the particular dog and how you raise him or her, they will generally be more or less energetic. This means that if you are more energetic and enjoy getting out for plenty of walks or play at the local park, your dog will grow up to enjoy these activities too. It's a simple formula: you are more energetic, your dog is more energetic and both of you will be healthier and happier.

I've had Dachshund clients whose dogs were calm, quiet, snoozy (and overweight), and others whose dogs loved getting outside and participating in highly energetic pursuits, so long as the weather was not too hot, cold or wet. In other words, if you're active, your dog most likely will be, too.

A healthy Dachshund will need to burn off their daily pent up energy by going for at least two to three good walks of 20 or 30 minutes each beside their human companions every day, plus have an opportunity to run free in the back yard chasing a ball or Frisbee, or playing and when properly socialized, this can include playing amidst other small dogs, in a secure off-leash area.

In order for this loving and loyal little dog to be happy and well balanced, they will want to be taken everywhere with you, which also helps to socialize, exercise their brains and prevent them from becoming bored, lazy or overweight.

Leaving a loving, affectionate dog alone for many hours every day that has been bred to be a canine companion, will be torture for them that could result in this dog becoming depressed, or making his or her own entertainment by becoming destructive and/or noisy by barking or howling all day.

The Dachshund, in order to maintain a healthy weight, will require daily moderate exercising. Keep in mind that if this dog is permitted to become lazy and inactive, they will quickly gain weight, which can contribute to future health issues. There are far too many fat Dachshunds in the world today.

A very good way to give this dog the amount of physical and mental exercise they really need is to teach them to perform simple tricks, or train them to run an Agility course. When well-socialized, a Dachshund with a reliable personality could also be a wonderful therapy dog for those living in care facilities that are missing having a dog as part of their life. Training your dog to visit care facilities can bring much joy, immediately light up lives and bring smiles to those who are otherwise having an uninteresting day.

Ideal Living Conditions for a Happy Dachshund

This affectionate companion is the perfect candidate for sharing life in a smaller, condominium or apartment-sized space, so long as you make the effort to ensure that they get outside for their disciplined, on-leash walks, play and socializing every day.

There is no doubt that whether you have a miniature or standard sized Dachshund, although lower to the ground than every other breed, this will be a companion with a loving personality that will require plenty of attention and being close to you throughout whatever you're doing in your day. To expect this dog to spend many hours alone every day could lead to him or her becoming a neurotic, excessive barker that certainly will not endear you to your neighbors.

"First, I want you to make sure that my dog is still in there someplace."

Also, keep in mind that while this amusing canine character can sometimes be stubborn (especially if they think the leadership role has defaulted to them), the personality of every Dachshund will be different and they will develop traits and quirks that are unique to each dog.

How each puppy will develop will depend upon the temperament of the parents, the environment where they are raised and how they are trained and socialized. The Dachshund is generally a curious, happy, intelligent, eager to please student that may enjoy, for instance, running an Agility course, Trick Training or Advanced Obedience. This dog will respond well to fair, fun and consistent training programs involving treat-based rewards or reinforcement.

Many guardians of this breed will agree that their comical little companions will faithfully follow them from room to room, as if attached by an invisible umbilical cord, because they just don't like to be left alone.

Properly socializing a Dachshund early on, during the first three months of his or her life, will greatly influence the dog's temperament, personality and behavior as he or she matures into adulthood. Continuing to shape the personality of the dog through adolescence and on into adulthood with proper socializing, training, adequate exercise, and firm rules and boundaries, will help to ensure a well-mannered dog.

You'll also find that it's very difficult to get upset with a dog that only wants to spend all of their time in your company, especially when they're gazing lovingly at you with those big pleading eyes and a sweet, soulful expression that could turn even the stoniest of hearts to mush.

If you are unable to commit to providing the proper routine for this dog on a daily basis, that includes on-going socialization, training, and spending the majority of his or her time in your company, this loving companion will very likely first become unhealthily overweight, and second, may easily become nervous, anxious and suffer from separation anxiety. A dog that is suffering in this way, unlike some other behavioral issues, can take much patience and a very long time to turn around.

An under-exercised dog will become fat, bored and unhappy, which can then cause them to develop behavioral problems that could include acting out in destructive ways by chewing *"off limits"* items in the home, digging holes in the garden, escaping the back yard, excessive barking, and ultimately suffering from anxiety and stress that can prematurely shorten their life.

In order to raise a happy Dachshund that will be a contented member of your family, it will be essential that you provide him or her with a moderate amount of daily disciplined walks and the opportunity for play time or learning a fun canine sport (where they get to use their mind), in order to maintain a happy disposition and a healthy weight.

 The best you can do for this companion is to properly train, socialize and exercise them every day beginning from the time when you first bring them home from the breeders.

 Above all else, never forget that all dogs (no matter their size) are pack animals, which means that it is not normal for them to spend long periods of time by themselves. This is even more important with a dog that used to be a busy, working hound, and now has become a more sedate family companion. Always remember that when you adopt a dog into your family you become their pack and you cannot simply abandon them when it's convenient for you to do so.

In other words, if you're planning to leave your companion alone for many hours every day, while you're at work or out for an evening at the pub with friends, don't get a Dachshund (or ANY dog for that matter); if you do, you will undoubtedly be contributing to your fur friend developing a depressed and unhappy state of mind, and where the Dachshund is concerned, most likely depression, nervousness that can lead to aggression, and the stress of separation anxiety.

As well, when a bored Dachshund has to find ways to entertain his or herself, you will also be opening the door to your loyal and affectionate dog developing unwanted behaviors. These behaviors can include becoming destructive, barking or whining and crying until they become hoarse, digging holes in the back yard, or attempting to escape so they can wander the neighborhood in search of their human guardian, that could lure them far away from home.

In a Nutshell

The bottom line here is that the Dachshund is usually an affectionate, loving, and playful, small companion that requires several short walks every day, plus the opportunity for off-leash play. This little dog may also enjoy learning new tricks and routines or canine sports, and the opportunity to socialize with other small dogs and people.

This Chapter also outlines several different canine sports that an energetic Dachshund may excel at, such as Agility, or Trick Training. Truly consider involving this dog in a sport, because this is a great way to provide them with the exercise they need in a disciplined way that will engage their mind and help to ensure that your dog remains a healthy and happy family member, while also teaching them that you are their leader.

TAKE AWAY TIP: While this dog usually needs a moderate amount of daily exercise, they also need maximum time in your company and will excel when you provide them with a daily routine that takes into consideration what is appropriate for their best physical and mental health.

Chapter 7: Feeding the Happy Dachshund

*"I feel sorry for people who don't have dogs.
I hear they have to pick up food they drop on the floor."*
— Unknown

It's not rocket science to grasp the concept that a properly fed Dachshund means a healthy, happy and longer-lived companion, so make sure that you spend an appropriate amount of time to research high-quality food and treats that will be the best for your happy Dachshund.

We are what we eat, and the same is absolutely true for our canine companions. Usually this breed will have a healthy appetite, however, any dog can develop picky eating habits, so make sure that you don't get into the habit of *"doctoring"* their food bowl with your human food. If you do, your dog may soon refuse to eat their doggy dinner. Don't worry, though, because even a picky eater will not starve him or herself, and if they refuse their expensive dog dinner tonight, so long as you don't cave, they WILL be hungry tomorrow.

First, remember that our canine friends are carnivores, which means that they derive their energy and nutrient requirements and maintain their health by consuming a diet consisting mainly or exclusively of the flesh of animal tissues. In other words, your dog is a meat eater.

Many dog owners underestimate the importance of feeding their dog a high-quality dog food and they make the mistake of shopping for dog food by price alone. The problem with this method is that the cheaper the dog food is, the poorer the quality. Inexpensive dog food brands use low-quality fillers and other ingredients to add bulk to the product, but these ingredients do not usually provide any nutritional benefit. Without a healthy, high-quality diet, your dog may not live as long as he or she could because poorly chosen food may lead to the development of health problems.

When choosing an appropriate diet for your Dachshund, considering the physiology of the canine's teeth, jaws and digestive tract will give you a better understanding of what food they should be eating.

Teeth, Jaws, and Digestive Tract

Teeth: canine teeth are all pointed because they are designed to rip, shred and tear into animal meat and bone. An adult dog has on average a third more teeth than his human guardian.

Adult canines have 42 permanent teeth in comparison to a measly 32 human teeth (without counting any wisdom teeth, which are "bonus"). Puppies have on average 28 baby teeth, while human babies will possess 20 "baby" teeth. Puppies start losing baby teeth at approximately 12 to 16 weeks of age. By four months of age, almost all of a puppy's baby teeth have been shed and many of the permanent teeth have already grown and are in place.

Jaws: every canine is born equipped with powerful jaws and neck muscles for the specific purpose of being able to pull down and tear apart their hunted prey.

The jaw of every canine opens widely to hold large pieces of meat and bone, while the actual mechanics of the canine jaw permits only vertical (up and down) movement that is designed for crushing.

Digestive Tract: the canine digestive tract is short, simple and designed to move their natural choice of food (hide, meat and bone) quickly through their systems.

We humans need vegetables and plant matter in our diet and have the flat molars to effectively crush and chew them. While we often believe our dogs require the same, when choosing an appropriate food source for your Dachshund, you need to consider that vegetables and

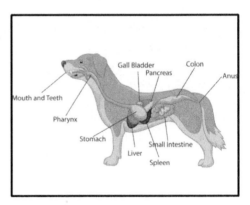

plant matter require more time to break down in the gastrointestinal tract. This in turn, requires a more complex digestive system that the canine body simply does not have.

The canine digestive system is unable to break down vegetable matter, which is why whole vegetables look pretty much the same going into your dog, as they do coming out the other end.

Consider how much healthier and longer-lived your beloved Dachshund can be if, instead of largely ignoring nature's design for our canine companions, we choose to feed them whole, unprocessed, species-appropriate food.

Whatever you decide to feed your dog, keep in mind that, just as too much wheat or other grains and fillers in our human diet are having detrimental effects on our human health, the same can be very true for our dogs.

Read the labels so that you can be certain to avoid foods that contain fillers or high amounts of grains, because these are inappropriate for a healthy canine diet.

Control of Your Happy Dachshund's Food

Some Dachshunds may be picky eaters, while others may have a moderately healthy appetite. This dog can also be quite possessive of their food. If he or she begins to show signs of defending their bowl with aggression, this behavior must be immediately nipped in the bud.

 Any dog can get bored with eating the same food every day, so mix it up a little. For instance, my dog, Boris, usually has little interest in food during the morning, but is ready for his dental treat at high noon. His internal clock is spot on and if I'm not paying attention to the time, he just calmly sits there staring at me until I get it.

It's important that your Dachshund understands that YOU are in control of their food source. Once they understand this, they will also figure out that there will be windows of opportunity for receiving and eating their food, and this routine will help to develop healthy eating habits.

Many people use a scoop or measuring cup to put dry food into their dog's bowl. This is a mistake, because it's very important to mix your dog's food with your hands, so that your scent is all over the food, before you give it to them to eat. This sends a "message" to your dog that you are their pack leader, because it mimics what would happen if you were the alpha dog out hunting for your food in the wild.

For instance, while a pack of wild dogs hunting for food all work hard to capture their prey, the alpha pack leader always gets to eat first while all the other dogs must wait until the leader of the pack eats their fill, before they can rush in to eat what is left over.

Therefore, when you are mixing your domesticated dog's dinner with your hands, you are sending them the subtle message that you're the pack leader, you've already eaten your fill and you are now allowing them to eat what was left over.

Nutritional Needs of the Dachshund

Before you go shopping for dog food take the time to learn the basics about the nutritional needs of your dog. Dogs are primarily carnivorous animals, which means that most of their nutritional needs should come from animal sources – including meat, fish, and eggs. Your dog needs a balance of protein and fat in their diet, plus healthy carbohydrates that can provide energy, fiber and other essential nutrients. It is important that your dog's daily food provides for their basic nutritional needs, because that is what he or she will be eating most of the time.

If you want to get into the specifics, know that protein is the most important nutrient for a dog and is required for healthy puppy growth and development. When your puppy grows up, protein will help him or her maintain lean muscle mass, so they do not become overweight or obese. Your puppy needs at least 22% protein in their diet and an adult dog needs 18%.

Next to protein, the most important nutrient for dogs is fat. While you may think of fat as a bad thing, it's actually an essential part of a balanced diet for dogs. Fat provides a concentrated source of energy and it helps your dog absorb and utilize fat-soluble vitamins. Fat should come from healthy animal sources such as chicken fat or salmon oil and should make up at least 8% of your young dog's diet. An adult dog will require a minimum of 5%.

Technically speaking, dogs do not have specific requirements for carbohydrate in their diet. Carbs can provide energy and they contain fibre as well as other nutrients.

What you also need to remember is that your dog's body is not optimized for digesting and absorbing nutrition from plant products as much as from animal products, which means that carbohydrates in your dog's diet should be limited. They should also come from easily digestible sources like whole grains, starchy vegetables, beans, or legumes.

Choosing a High-Quality Dog Food Brand

When shopping for food for your Dachshund, you need to take the time to carefully read the information on the package so that you can determine the quality of the product.

Also, if you're going to make comparisons between different products, there are three specific things to look for on the label.

AAFCO Statement of Nutritional Adequacy

First, look for the Association of American Feed Control Officials (AAFCO) statement of nutritional adequacy. This is an organization that sets and upholds standards for pet food and animal feed. If you and your dog live in the UK, check for information from the Food Standards Agency (FSA).

Before a product hits the shelf, these organizations examine it to make sure it meets the minimum nutritional requirements for the intended animal, which, in this case, is your dog. If the product is nutritionally balanced for dogs, you will see a statement like this somewhere on the label:

"[Product Name] is formulated to meet the nutritional levels established by the AAFCO Dog Food Nutrient Profiles."

If you see this on the package, you can rest assured that it will meet your dog's minimum nutritional needs. Keep in mind, however, that the AAFCO statement does not guarantee quality – you still have to read the ingredients list noted on the package to determine whether the product is any good or not.

Guaranteed Analysis

After the AAFCO statement, look at the guaranteed analysis – this tells you the percentages of protein, fat, fibre and moisture in the product. You can use the guaranteed analysis to make a direct comparison between products using those minimum values from the last section. Because your dog is better able to digest meat than plant foods, try to keep the fibre content under 5%.

Ingredients List

After checking the guaranteed analysis, the final place to look is the ingredients list.

The ingredients list is ordered in descending order by volume, which means that the ingredients at the top of the list are used in the highest quantity – this is the same for packages of food that you eat. You will want to see healthy, high-quality ingredients at the beginning of the list starting with a source of animal protein. Dogs are carnivores, which means that their bodies are better able to digest and absorb nutrition from animal sources. Quality sources of animal protein for dogs include poultry, meat, and seafood.

Aside from proteins, fats, and carbohydrates, there are some other beneficial ingredients you can look for. Supplemental vitamins and minerals can improve your dog's health, because they help to ensure that your dog's specific nutritional needs are met.

DID YOU KNOW? *Synthetic supplements are not as good for your dog as natural sources for the same nutrients – things like fresh fruits and vegetables. When it comes to mineral supplements, chelated minerals are ideal – these are minerals that have been bound to protein molecules, which makes them easier for your dog's body to utilize. If you see "dried fermentation products" on the list, do not be alarmed – these are probiotics that can support your dog's digestion.*

Feeding Tips

- Feeding amounts for canines vary based on factors such as breed, lifestyle, and body condition.

- While feeding suggestions are provided on all dog food packaging, your vet may be the best resource for telling you exactly how much you should be feeding your dog. See next section for generic feeding amount guidelines.

- Consult your vet regularly about your puppy's weight as achieving and maintaining an ideal weight not only reduces many health risks, but can also help your puppy have a more energetic, longer and healthier life.

- Do not overfeed! Numerous studies showed that dogs whose diets were responsibly restricted early on experienced longer lifespans and later onset of problems like osteoarthritis.

- If you give your dog the occasional treat or if you use treats for training, always remember to take this into account and reduce the daily food allowance.

- As a rule of thumb, treats shouldn't make up more than 10% of your dog's daily calorie intake as this can unbalance his diet.

- Although it's tempting and convenient to feed your puppy table scraps, they do not provide your pup with the correct balance of nutrients.

- A puppy or adult dog rarely says no to food, but that does not mean they are always hungry. Constantly giving them food can lead to unwanted behavior problems such as "begging for food" and hyper activity whenever they see you eating. Dogs are hard wired to always be foraging and looking for food and no matter how much you feed them, they will still ask for more. Therefore, make sure you don't let them develop this bad habit of begging for food.

❧ Any time you change your dog's diet, be sure to mix a little of the old food with the new food to transition them slowly – this will help to prevent digestive upset.

❧ If you mix your dog's food properly and he or she is still having digestive issues, it could be something else – such as food allergies.

❧ Food allergies affect dogs in a different way than they affect humans. While you might feel nauseous or sick after eating something you are allergic to, your dog will be more likely to develop skin problems, or throw up what they just ate.

❧ Red, itchy, and inflamed skin is a common sign of food allergies.

❧ Technically, your dog can develop an allergy to any food he or she eats, but there are some ingredients more likely to trigger food allergies in dogs than others.

❧ Some of the most common food allergens for dogs include beef, chicken, dairy, lamb, fish, corn, eggs, wheat, and soy, and this is usually because they came from food sources that are not "clean" or "organic". For instance, unless the chosen food is certified organic, grass fed and contains no additives, there are hidden components that can cause allergic responses. Crops such as corn, soy or wheat are often sprayed with chemicals and fed to farmed animals to fatten them up. This means that your dog may not be allergic to beef, but may be allergic to the wheat, soy or corn that's been fed to the animals.

❀ If you suspect that your Dachshund has a food allergy, you may need to put him or her on an elimination diet for 12 weeks or until all signs of the allergy have disappeared. At that point you can either keep feeding the elimination diet or switch to a food that doesn't contain the allergen.

Feeding Puppies

A general rule of thumb for growing Dachshund puppies is to feed daily amounts of between 2 and 3% of what the puppy's adult weight is projected to be or 10% of the puppy's current body weight. You will want to keep in mind that while all puppies require extra protein during the first two years of their life to help them develop into healthy adult dogs, this is especially important with higher energy puppies.

You will also want to keep a close eye to make sure that this small puppy is eating and drinking enough throughout the day. Setting regular feeding times each day is especially important with smaller puppies.

There are now many foods on the market that are formulated for all stages of a dog's life (including the puppy stage). Whether you choose one of these foods or a food specially formulated for early stages of growth, puppies will need to be fed smaller meals more frequently throughout the day (between 3 and 5 times), until they are at least one year of age.

 Dachshunds can be considered adults after about a year. They may still be growing after this time, but at the 12-month mark you can start feeding your dog adult food.

Feeding Adults

Choose foods that list high-quality meat protein as the main ingredient and, depending on your dog's particular energy level, feed between 2 and 3% of their body weight every day. While some dogs prefer one meal a day, most will appreciate morning food (after a walk) and evening food (after a walk).

Be careful not to get caught up in "convenience" when you are out grocery shopping for yourself, and decide to buy your Dachshund's food at the same place, because most grocery stores tend to carry inferior brands of dog food.

Instead, make the time to visit your local pet store, talk with educated representatives, avoid grains, and choose quality sources of meat protein for healthy puppies and dogs, including beef, buffalo, chicken, duck, fish, hare, lamb, ostrich, pork, rabbit, turkey, venison, or any other source of wild meaty protein.

Treats

There are endless choices of dog treats lining the shelves of every feed store, pet store, and grocery store, and it will be an overwhelming task to choose wisely, unless you keep one simple rule in mind, and choose treats that contain only one ingredient or very few ingredients.

Whatever reason you choose to give treats to your Dachshund, keep in mind that if we treat our dogs too often throughout the day, they can become overweight, and we may create a picky eater who will no longer want to eat their regular meals. Think about it – if you got to eat only your favourite tasty treats throughout the day, would you be excited about consuming a less flavourful meal come dinner time?

DID YOU KNOW? *Researchers in Sweden have discovered that dogs were happier when they had to <u>earn</u> their treats as a reward for completing a task, rather than just being given a treat for looking cute, because just like us humans who get that happy "eureka" moment when we finally solve a problem, the same is true for our canine counterparts. The Dachshund is usually food motivated, which makes him or her the perfect dog for positive training methods that involve treat reinforcement.*

Dangerous Treats

Always carefully read labels and take note of where treats are manufactured, because not all countries have the most stringent manufacturing protocols, and honestly there are many treats that you absolutely should NOT be feeding your dog, including:

Rawhide, which is soaked in an ash/lye solution to remove every particle of meat, fat and hair and then further soaked in bleach to remove remaining traces of the ash/lye solution. Now that the product is no longer food, it no longer has to comply with food regulations.

The wet rawhide is shaped into chews, and once dry it shrinks to approximately 25% of its original size before arsenic-based products are used as preservatives, and antibiotics and insecticides are added to kill bacteria.

While rawhide chews are tough and long lasting, when a dog chews a rawhide treat, they ingest many harsh chemicals. Also, when your dog swallows a piece of rawhide, that piece can swell up to four times its size inside your dog's stomach, which can cause anything from mild to severe gastric blockages that could become life threatening and require surgery. As much as it might be convenient for you to be able to give your dog or puppy a treat that will occupy them for a considerable time, if it's rawhide, just say "No".

Pig's Ears are very attractive to most dogs that will eagerly devour them, and they're "natural" because they're ears, so what could be wrong? Actually, these are thin, crispy and very high in fat, which can cause stomach upsets, vomiting and diarrhoea. In addition, pieces can break off and become stuck in a dog's throat.

Also, pig ears are often processed and preserved with unhealthy chemicals that discerning dog guardians will not want to feed their dogs. Just say "No".

Hoof Treats are actual cow, horse and pig hooves that humans believe are healthy, *"natural"* treat choices for their dogs when the truth is that after processing with harsh chemicals, preservatives and antibiotics, they retain little, if any, of their *"natural"* qualities.

Also, hooves are very hard and can cause the chipping or breaking of your dog's teeth as well as perforation or blockages in your dog's intestines. Just say "No".

Healthy Treats

There are so many healthy treat choices available, which means that there is no excuse for feeding your Dachshund unhealthy, nutrient-deficient treats that could harm them. Read the labels to make sure the treats you are choosing are appropriately sized for your dog and are of the highest quality. Examples of healthy treats include:

Hard Treats: come in many varieties of shapes, sizes and flavors and will help to keep your dog's teeth cleaner.

Soft Treats: are also available in endless varieties and flavors, suitable for all the different needs of our furry friends and are often smaller in size and used for training purposes.

Dental Treats or Chews: are designed with the specific purpose of helping your dog to maintain healthy teeth and gums by exercising the jaw and massaging gums, while removing plaque build-up near the gum line.

The best thing you can do for your dog's oral hygiene is to brush his teeth. However, dog dental chews are an excellent top-up between brushes or for dogs who will not let you get anywhere near their teeth without a great struggle. Dental chews come in both edible and non-edible varieties and lots of dogs love the taste of edible chews and think of them as a tasty treat. Non-edible chews are a bit like toys for many dogs and satisfy their natural urge to chew.

Freeze-Dried and Jerky Treats: offer a tasty morsel most dogs find irresistible as they are usually made of simple, meaty ingredients, such as liver, poultry and seafood. Be careful when choosing jerky treats, as they are often processed with too much salt.

Human Food Treats: be very careful when feeding human foods to dogs as treats, because many of our foods contain unhealthy additives, such as salt, sugar and other ingredients that could be toxic and harmful.

Also, educate yourself about the common human foods that are actually poisonous to our canine friends, such as grapes, raisins, onions and chocolate, to name a few.

Generally, the treats you feed your dog should not make up more than approximately 10% of their daily food intake, so make sure the treats you choose are high quality, with single or few ingredients so that you can help to keep your Dachshund both happy and healthy.

The Right Food for Your Happy Dachshund

"Dog Food" has significantly changed since1785, when the English Sportman's Dictionary described the best diet for a dog's health in an

article entitled *"Dog"*. This article indicated that the best food for a dog was something called *"Greaves"*, described as "*the sediment of melted tallow made into cakes for dogs' food*".

From these meager beginnings, commercially manufactured dog food has become a massively lucrative industry that has only fairly recently evolved beyond feeding our dogs the dregs of human leftovers, because it was cheap and convenient for us.

Even today, the majority of dog food choices often have far more to do with being convenient for humans to store and serve, than it does with being a diet truly designed to be a nutritionally balanced, healthy food choice for our canine companions.

Educating yourself by talking to experts and reading everything you can find on the subject, plus taking into consideration several relevant factors, will help to answer the dog food question for you and your dog.

For instance, where you live may dictate what sorts of foods you have access to, while other factors to consider will include the particular requirements of your dog, such as their age, energy and activity levels.

Our dogs are also suffering from many of the same life-threatening diseases that are commonly found in our human society (heart disease, cancer, diabetes, obesity). These diseases all have a direct correlation with over-feeding and/or eating genetically altered foods that are no longer pure, in favor of a convenient, processed and packaged diet that is quick and easy for us to serve.

The Raw Diet: raw feeding advocates believe that the ideal diet for

their dog is one which would be very similar to what a dog living in the wild would have access to while hunting or foraging.

These canine guardians are often opposed to feeding their dog any sort of commercially manufactured pet foods, because they consider them to be poor substitutes, and for the most part, I would agree.

For instance, many guardians of high energy, working breed dogs will agree that their dogs thrive on a raw or BARF (Biologically Appropriate Raw Food) diet and strongly believe that the potential benefits of feeding a raw dog food diet are many, whether your dog is earning a daily working wage or simply being your loyal companion, including:

- Healthy, shiny coats
- Decreased shedding
- Fewer allergy problems
- Healthier skin
- Cleaner teeth
- Fresher breath
- Increased energy levels
- Improved digestion
- Smaller stools
- Strengthened immune system
- Increased mobility in arthritic pets
- Increase or improvement in overall health

A raw diet is a direct evolution of what dogs ate before they became our domesticated pets and we turned toward commercially prepared, easy-to-serve dry dog food that required no special storage or preparation.

The Dehydrated Diet: is available in both raw and cooked meat forms, which are usually air dried to reduce moisture and inhibit bacterial growth. While the appearance of dehydrated dog food is very similar to dry kibble, the typical feeding methods include adding warm water before serving, which makes this type of diet both healthy for our dogs and convenient for us to serve.

Dehydrated recipes are made from minimally processed fresh, whole foods to create a healthy and nutritionally balanced meal that retains more of the overall nutritional value, and will meet or exceed the dietary requirements of a healthy canine.

A dehydrated diet is a convenient way to feed your dog a nutritious diet, because all you have to do is add warm water and wait five minutes while the food re-hydrates so your dog can enjoy a warm meal.

The Kibble Diet: there is no mistaking that the convenience and relative economy of dry dog food kibble, which had its beginnings in the 1940's, continues to be the most popular pet food choice for many dog-friendly humans. Thankfully, there are now many high-quality kibble foods available.

The Right Bowl for the Dachshund: there are many different types and categories of dog bowls, including Automatic Watering, Elevated, Ceramic, Stoneware, No Skid, No Tip, Slow Feeder, Stainless, Wooden and Travel Bowls.

Always purchase bowls that are appropriately sized for your particular dog, and consider an elevated dining table so that their head is up from the floor when eating and drinking.

Also, if your dog tends to eat too quickly, since they can suffer from bloat, you may want to consider a slow-feeder type of bowl to help slow them down.

In a Nutshell

While food and treat choices for your favorite furry Dachshund can be overwhelming, a basic understanding of canine physiology and making wise decisions concerning all the many different types of food and treats available, will help you to add many healthy and happy years to your dog's life.

You are the sole protector of your canine companion, and I cannot stress strongly enough the importance of a well thought out choice when deciding what brand and type of food and treats you will feed your loyal canine companion.

Appropriate food/treat choices and being careful to not overfeed, may not only increase the length of your dog's life by avoiding unwanted health conditions, such as obesity, high blood pressure or bladder stones, good food choices will also provide your dog with optimal health so they can feel good and live a happy life!

Chapter 8: Care of the Happy Dachshund

"When you adopt a dog, you have a lot of
very good days, and one very bad day."
— W. Bruce Cameron

Imagine you're travelling by car on a daily basis without being protected by a seatbelt or an airbag. How safe would you feel? Unfortunately, this is the reality for far too many of our furry friends, because their guardians have neglected their safety responsibilities.

NOTE: far too many humans are guilty of allowing their tiny canine travel companions to sit on their lap when they're driving. DO NOT get into this very dangerous habit. If you get into an accident, while the airbag may save your life, the force of it will probably kill the small dog sitting on your lap.

Now, imagine going for months without washing your hair, cutting your nails or brushing your teeth. Again, that is the reality for many dogs, because their owners have not been advised with respect to the importance of good grooming. How happy and well-behaved do you think such an ill cared for dog would be?

The following few paragraphs outline safe travelling, licensing, insurance and grooming requirements, all of which can help to ensure that your Dachshund is safe, legal and better cared for at the vet's office.

Keep in mind that if your dog is safely secured when travelling, they might not be dead or seriously injured should you be involved in a vehicle accident. We humans wear seatbelts to be safe – what about safety for our best fur friends?

Further, if your dog is properly licensed, they will be returned to you should they go missing, and this is a much happier dog than one spending who knows how long behind bars at a rescue or SPCA.

As well, if you have pet health insurance, chances are that your dog will be better cared for at the vet's office, which means a healthier and happier companion.

Tips for Keeping Your Dog Safe

Not So Safe Harness Restraints: is your canine companion safe when buckled into a safety harness for travel in vehicles? Be aware that many of the dog harnesses in the marketplace have a 100% failure rate.

If you cannot find a safety harness that is actually been strength tested and crash tested (i.e. optimal choice), the safest travel arrangement for any dog is to secure them inside a kennel, that is bolted to the floor or secured with the vehicle's seatbelt. Remember that a dog travelling in the front passenger seat, even one secured with a proper safety harness, may still sustain injuries (and even death) if the 100 mph force of the airbag strikes them.

Kennels: a dog kennel or crate will easily fit on the back seat of most vehicles and can be secured with the vehicle's restraint system. A Dachshund riding inside a kennel that is secure inside your vehicle will have the best protection in the case of a rollover accident, plus you will avoid the fines some locations are now levying for allowing a dog to roam freely inside a moving vehicle.

Air Travel: the Dachshund puppy will be small enough to fit into a soft Sherpa bag for travel inside an airplane cabin (as carry-on baggage), and some, depending on their size, may remain small enough to travel as carry-on luggage inside the airplane cabin when they are fully grown. Any standard-sized dogs that are too large to fit comfortably inside a Sherpa travel bag will need to be transported inside a heated cargo hold.

Licensing: when you purchase your dog a yearly license or identifying tag, they will be legal, and should they become lost when wearing a license, there is a much higher possibility that your dog will be returned to you, instead of spending their last few days behind bars at the local SPCA or rescue facility.

Pet Health Insurance: purchasing health insurance for your dog means that they will usually live a longer, healthier and happier life, because they will receive better care throughout their lifetime.

Be aware that you need to begin insurance when your dog is a young puppy, because waiting until they are older will mean that your monthly premiums are considerably higher.

Puppy Proofing

As a dog owner, it is your responsibility to make sure that your Dachshund's needs are taken care of. It all starts with prepping your home for a new puppy by puppy-proofing to keep your puppy safe. Next, you will need to learn what to feed your puppy and when to transition him to an adult dog food formula (previous chapter). You will also need to take care of your dog's grooming requirements, which is discussed later on in this chapter.

When it comes to preparing your home for a new dog, you will need to do some puppy-proofing. Start by walking through your home and try to view it through a puppy's eyes to identify potential dangers. Here's a list of some of the things you may need to do:

- ❧ Store cleaning products where your puppy cannot reach them or put them in a locked cabinet.

- ❧ Put all trash in a can with a tight-fitting lid or keep it secured in a cupboard.

- ❧ Store open food containers in your pantry or cupboards – anything left out needs a lid.

- ❧ Tie up or bundle any electrical cords and blind cords so your puppy cannot chew on them.

- ❧ Pick up small objects from the floor – they are a choking hazard for dogs.

- ❧ Cover open bodies of water (such as the toilet, bathtub, outdoor ponds, swimming pools, etc.).

- ❧ Put all medications and other toiletries where your puppy cannot reach them, such as in the medicine cabinet and use child-proof bottles.

- ❧ Make sure none of your houseplants or plants in your yard are toxic to dogs – if there are any suspect plants or flowers, remove them, move them out of reach, or fence them off.

- ❧ Keep your windows and doors securely closed when your puppy is out – use baby gates or pet gates to keep them away from areas where you do not want them to wander.

- ❧ If you have a cat, keep the litter box where your puppy cannot reach it, so he does not eat the clumps.

- 🐾 Dispose of all food waste properly so your puppy cannot get it – this is especially important for chicken bones and foods that are harmful to dogs.

- 🐾 Store all lawn and garden tools where your puppy cannot get to them and make sure they will not fall over if your puppy bumps into them.

- 🐾 If you have a yard, consider adding a fence to keep your puppy in.

- 🐾 Avoid using toxic chemical fertilizers, pesticides, or herbicides anywhere your puppy could be exposed.

Once you have puppy-proofed your home, the next step is to set up your puppy's area. You can choose a small room or use a puppy playpen to cordon off a section of a larger room. Place your puppy's crate and dog bed in the area as well as their food and water bowls and their toys. You will want to put your puppy in this area when you cannot actively watch him or her so they are less likely to get into trouble. While your puppy is very young, when you cannot closely watch them, you may want to confine him or her to their crate until they are housetrained.

Grooming Your Dog

Regular grooming is important for a happy and healthy Dachshund, because it keeps them clean, and their skin moisturized and bug free, plus grooming time can alert you to any problems before they become more serious. Especially for longer-haired dogs, it will also be a good idea to commit to at least a weekly brushing to remove debris and any tangled or matted hair.

Hair Brushing Technique

- 🐾 Use a wire-pin brush or a soft bristle brush to brush out your dog's coat at least twice a week.

- ❧ Start at the base of the neck and work your way down the back and sides, always brushing in the direction of hair growth.

- ❧ Next, brush down each leg then have your dog roll over so you can brush out their underside. Don't forget the tail if your dog has one..

- ❧ If you happen to find a snag, work through it gently with your fingers, so you do not cause painful hair pulling that can hurt your dog.

Depending upon whether you decide to fully groom your dog yourself, or will take him or her to the local doggy spa, you will require minimal equipment to keep the coat of your happy Dachshund looking his or her best. If you're just keeping on top of weekly brushing, all you will need is a soft bristle brush, and perhaps a flea comb (just in case). If you're planning to do all your dog's grooming yourself, see *"Grooming Equipment You Will Need"* on the next page.

Also, you will want to get your dog used to their grooming routine early on, because otherwise, every time your dog needs to be bathed or brushed will end up being a traumatic experience for both dog and human that can last for many years. Start them off right so you can both enjoy grooming time.

 I've been asked to groom dogs that have been kicked out of every grooming salon because their owners did not take the time to introduce the puppy to bath time, nail clipping and other necessary grooming procedures at a young age.

I can tell you from much personal experience that having to groom a writhing, screaming dog that is all teeth, because they are fighting the procedure, is hell on wheels, and the very worst case I ever encountered

was with a dog weighing only 4 pounds (1.8 kg). Try going through this with an unwilling Dachshund, and you will very soon be wishing your companion were a chia pet.

Grooming Equipment You Will Need

A standard arsenal of equipment for the DIY groomer that will help you keep your dog looking their best will include the following:

Bristle brush – is the ideal tool for removing debris minimal mats from the Dachshund's coat, while at the same time distributing natural oils to keep the coat looking healthy and shiny.

Sturdy Metal Comb – get one that has rotating teeth as this pulls the hair much less.

Slicker Brush – this has rows of metal teeth placed closely together and is a great tool for smoothing the coat.

Nail clippers or a slow speed pet Dremel™ – will be tools you need to use every couple of weeks or more, depending on how quickly your dog's nails grow and what types of surfaces they may be walking on. The pet Dremel is perfect for smoothing the sharp edges that nail clippers leave, and if you are vigilant with regular use of the Dremel, you may never have to clip.

Flea comb – hopefully you won't ever need one, however, as the name suggests, these combs are designed for the specific purpose of removing fleas from a dog's coat. Usually small in size for manoeuvring in tight spaces, they may be made of plastic or metal with the teeth of the comb placed very close together to trap hiding fleas.

Tick Twister – hopefully your dog won't ever get a tick, but if they do, this is a simple device for painlessly, easily and quickly removing ticks that have imbedded themselves in your dog's skin.

Grooming Products You Will Need

Products you will need to invest in when bathing your dog yourself will include shampoos, conditioners, creams, lotions, sprays and powders.

Shampoos: NEVER make the mistake of using human shampoo or conditioner that has a pH balance of 5.5, for bathing your dog. Our canine companions have an almost neutral pH balance of 7.5, and any shampoo with a lower pH will be harmful to your dog, because it will strip the natural oils and be too harshly acidic for their coat and skin, which can create itchy skin problems and allow for a very unhappy dog.

Conditioners: taking the extra time to condition your dog's coat will not only make it look and feel better, it will also add additional benefits, including:

- Preventing the escape of natural oils and moisture
- Keeping the coat cleaner for a longer period of time
- Repairing a coat that has become dull, damaged or dry
- Restoring a soft, silky feel
- Helping the coat dry more quickly
- Protecting from the heat of the dryer and breakage of hair

The benefits of spending the extra two minutes to condition your dog's coat will be appreciated by both yourself and your dog that will have overall healthy, moisturized skin and a coat with a natural shine.

Bathing your dog:

- ❧ To bathe your dog, simply fill your bathtub with a few inches of lukewarm water and place your dog in it – you can put a bath mat or towel down to keep him from slipping.

- ❧ Then, use a cup or a hand sprayer to wet down your dog's coat and work a little bit of dog-friendly shampoo into a thick lather.

- ❧ Rinse the coat well until the coat is completely free of all of the shampoo suds, squeeze out the excess water and then towel your dog dry.

- ❧ Unless your dog gets dirty, you should only plan to bathe him once every 4 to 6 weeks, because bathing too often can dry out your dog's skin and coat.

<u>Oops, My Dog Has Fleas</u>

You haven't been paying attention and now realize that your dog is suffering from an infestation of fleas. Now is the time to bathe them with shampoo containing pyrethrum (a botanical extract found in small, white daisies) or a shampoo containing citrus or tea tree oil.

Also, you can bathe and spray them with the non-toxic and highly effective CedarCide products, which can also be used to spray down their bedding and any carpets in the home, and will kill fleas (or other crawly creatures) on contact without harming anyone.

CedarCide is a company that makes 100% safe, organic products to control biting bugs on your furry friends without worrying about harmful chemicals that are not good for you, your children or your canine companions.

Simply spray it on and bugs of any sort that come into contact with the solution will be dead, while your dog's coat will be shiny and fresh smelling, like the inside of a cedar chest.

Nail Care

Many canine guardians neglect taking proper care of their dog's toenails, which can lead to many problems later in life, such as painful joints and difficulty walking, which will make for a very unhealthy and unhappy dog.

Purchase a good pair of medium-sized, scissor-type nail clippers with a safety stop and learn how to properly use them. If you don't, your dog's nails will soon be too long and the vein inside the nail will also grow too long and you will be unable to keep them as short as they should be.

Depending on the types of surfaces your Dachshund is walking on, you should plan to clip your dog's nails approximately every two weeks. When trimming the nails, be sure to only snip the tip, so you do not accidentally cut into the vein, which will be painful and will cause your dog to bleed.

Steps For Nail Clipping

* Hold your canine's paw firmly but gently.

* Trim the nail below the quick at a 45° angle, cutting small amounts at a time.

* Trim until you reach the white inside the nail with a small black dot at the centre. If you can't see the white, you can cut a bit more.

 If your puppy has not had their "dew claws" removed (these are the claws that are on the side of the foot that never touch the ground), they still continue to grow. If you

miss clipping these nails, they will soon grow into a circle that will be very difficult to clip and can even grow back into the dog's leg causing great pain.

Styptic Powder: you will always want to avoid causing any pain when trimming your Dachshund's toenails, because you don't want to destroy their trust in you regularly performing this necessary task.

However, accidents do happen, therefore if you clip too short, and accidentally cut into the vein in the toenail, know that you will cause your dog pain, and that the toenail will bleed. Therefore, it is always a good idea to keep some styptic powder (often called *"Kwik Stop"*) in your grooming kit.

Dip a moistened finger into the powder and apply it with pressure to the end of the bleeding nail, because this is the quickest way to stop a nail from bleeding in just a few seconds.

Some dogs prefer having their nails trimmed with a rotary "Dremel" type of device that grinds down the excess nail. With this tool, it is easier to avoid cutting into the vein, and if you use this tool every week, you can trim shorter and will never have to actually clip the nails.

 Keep in mind that if you decide to trim your dog's nails this way, you MUST purchase a "doggy Dremel" made especially for this purpose, because using your shop Dremel will harm your dog's nails as it is too high speed and will burn the nails.

Ear Care

Dogs can often suffer from painful ear infections, because the ears can easily retain moisture.

Paying attention and keeping your dog's ears clean and dry will prevent this type of unhappy pain and suffering. Make sure that you keep ear powders and cleaning solutions in your grooming kit, because with proper preventative care, your dog need never suffer from an ear infection.

Ear Powders: which can be purchased at any pet store, are designed to help keep your dog's ears dry while at the same time inhibiting the growth of bacteria that can lead to infections. Ear powders are also used when removing excess hair growth from inside a dog's ear canal, as the powder makes it easier to grip the hair.

Ear Cleaning Solutions: your local pet store will offer a wide variety of ear cleaning creams, drops, oils, rinses or wipes specially formulated for cleaning your Dachshund's ears.

In addition, there are many home remedies that will just as efficiently clean your dog's ears without the high price tag, including Witch Hazel (a 50:50 solution of Organic Apple Cider Vinegar and Purified Water) or a 50:50 solution of Hydrogen Peroxide and Purified Water.

Cleaning your dog's ears

- ☙ Lift your dog's ear, holding it between your thumb and forefinger to get a good look inside the ear.

- ☙ Check for redness, discharge or bad smell. It is normal to see a small amount of light-coloured wax. If there is a very large amount, the ears are red, or there appears to be pus or a bad smell, this is a sign of a problem that will require immediate veterinary attention.

- ☙ Gently wipe around the entrance of the ear canal with damp cotton wool, removing dirt or excess wax.

- ☙ Insert the tip of the bottle into the ear canal making sure not to insert it too far, and then squeeze the bottle to release the ear cleaner.

- ❈ Massage the base of the ear to help the cleaner pass inside the ear canal.

- ❈ Wipe away any excess cleaner amount with damp cotton wool.

- ❈ Repeat the same process for the other ear.

- ❈ If your vet has prescribed ear drops to use, it's best to apply them straight after you've finished cleaning the ears. This will ensure that the medicine will enter the ear effectively and be absorbed without being blocked by excess wax.

Teeth Care

Another greatly overlooked area in your happy Dachshund's health is ensuring that their teeth are clean and properly looked after, so that they don't suffer from loose or broken teeth, and plaque build-up that leads to painful gum disease. You know how miserable a toothache can be – imagine your poor dog that cannot tell you how unhappy they are.

Many guardians use the excuse that *"my dog doesn't like it"* when they try to brush their dog's teeth, and overlook the fact that in order to keep their entire dog healthy, they <u>must</u> have healthy teeth and the only way to ensure this, is to commit to making the time to brush your dog's teeth every day.

Canine Toothpastes: are flavoured with beef or chicken in an attempt to appeal to the dog's taste buds, while some contain baking soda, which is the same mild abrasive found in many human pastes, and are designed to gently scrub the teeth.

Other types of canine toothpastes are formulated with enzymes that are designed to work chemically by breaking down tartar or plaque in the dog's mouth. While these pastes don't need to be washed off your dog's teeth and are safe for them to swallow, whether or not they remain on the dog's teeth long enough to do any good might be debatable.

Just as effective for killing germs, whitening and cleaning your dog's teeth, and much less expensive than fancy pastes, is old-fashioned hydrogen peroxide; you can also combine hydrogen peroxide (3% food grade), Aloe Vera juice (1:1) with a little bit of baking soda.

How can I brush my dog's teeth?

In the beginning, it is important to get your dog used to the toothpaste and to the whole brushing experience. Here is the technique I use:

- Check your dog's teeth and gums often to see what is normal so you can spot any issues or problems.

- During the first few days, hold your dog as you would normally when you are petting him or her.

- Gently stroke the outside of the cheeks with your finger for 1 or 2 minutes.

- After each session, reward your dog with praise and a treat they like. For the next few days, after your dog has become comfortable with this activity, place a small amount of toothpaste on your finger and let your dog try the flavour.

- Next, you should introduce your dog to a canine toothbrush or finger brush.

- Apply a pea-sized amount of toothpaste that has been specially formulated for dogs on the brush. Gently lift your dog's upper lip and place the brush against an upper tooth.

- With a slow circular motion, brush gently only that tooth and the adjoining gum line.

- ❧ Every following day gradually increase the number of teeth being brushed. Remember to go slowly, do not continue beyond your dog's point of comfort.

- ❧ Build up to 30 seconds of brushing per side.

- ❧ The easiest way to do this is to go straight, pushing the brush gently from front to back along the gumline. Next, add in the gentle circular motion.

- ❧ You do not have to brush the inside of the teeth, as the tongue keeps that side relatively free of plaque.

- ❧ After each session reward your dog with a treat and lots of praise.

- ❧ Ideally, brushing should be done daily, but if you miss 1-2 days per week, that would not be a big concern.

The easiest and most effective way to brush a dog's teeth is with an electric toothbrush (the rotary type) that does all the work for you. You can easily slowly introduce this method, just as you did with the manual brush, and once your dog gets used to the buzzing, all you have to do is hold the brush against their teeth.

Paw Care

If your dog runs over sharp barnacles on the beach, jogs with you on hard road surfaces, or over other rough terrain, this can cause cuts and scrapes and very rough surfaces on the paws. If you live in a hot climate, be aware that sidewalks, road surfaces and sandy beaches can get extremely hot for your dog's feet.

Paw Creams: depending upon activity levels and the types of surfaces our canine counterparts usually walk on, they may suffer from cracked or rough pads. You can restore resiliency and keep your dog's paws
in healthy condition by regularly applying a cream or lotion to protect

their paw pads. A good time to do this is just after you've clipped their nails.

In a Nutshell

Learning about simple steps that will keep your Dachshund safe, and what's involved in keeping him or her properly groomed will go a long way toward helping them to live a long, happy and healthy life.

While for many people the concept of grooming a dog conjures up notions of brushes and bows, it is in fact a vital element to their overall health and wellbeing.

Regularly grooming your dog will help you detect any underlying diseases or conditions early and will allow your beloved fur friend to feel better and live a longer and happier life.

Chapter 9: Are YOU the Ideal Happy Dachshund Guardian?

"A dog is the only thing on earth that loves you more than he loves himself."
— Josh Billings

If you have not chosen wisely when sharing your life with a canine companion, you are setting yourself, your family, your friends and your neighbours up for many years of stress, guilt and unhappiness.

It is vitally important that you take a good hard look at your own energy level and lifestyle, ask yourself some serious questions that you honestly answer, and not scrimp on taking the time to do plenty of research about the breed of dog you may be considering.

Sharing your life with a canine friend should never be undertaken lightly, or on a whim or spur of the moment decision, or because you like the colour of a dog's coat or the sweet expression on their face.

Before you can learn how to become your dog's ideal guardian, you need to first have no doubt in your mind that you have the energy, commitment, time and skill level necessary to raise a happy dog. Once this is established in the affirmative, you then need to know how to choose the right breed of puppy or dog.

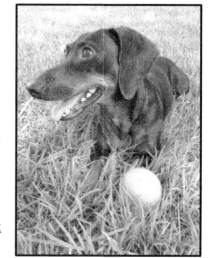

Choosing the <u>right</u> puppy for your family and your lifestyle is more important than you might imagine, and far too many people forget to consider how important is to choose a puppy or dog based on compatibility with their own energy and lifestyle.

For instance, many humans choose a puppy (or older dog) for all the <u>wrong</u> reasons, including because:

- 🐾 they like what it looks like

- 🐾 the breed may currently be popular

- 🐾 the breed appeared on TV or in a movie they enjoyed

- 🐾 their parents had the same kind of dog when they were a child

- 🐾 a friend has the same breed

- 🐾 they feel sorry for a homeless dog

- 🐾 a friend or family member can no longer keep their dog

- 🐾 the children are begging for a dog

- 🐾 someone was selling puppies on a street corner

While some of these above reasons can be honourable, the most important reasons for choosing to share your life with a particular canine companion has not been properly considered.

In order to make an intelligent choice that will bring happiness to everyone, you need to take a serious look at your life as it is today and also how you envision it to be during the next ten to fifteen years, and then ask yourself several very important questions, including:

Activity – Do I lead a highly active, medium or low-intensity life? For instance, am I out jogging the streets every morning, hiking local mountains or riding my bicycle five miles to the local grocery store? Does my job keep me away from home, and does my leisure time activity keep me in front of the computer or on the couch watching movies?

Travel – Do I travel a lot for work or pleasure? If you do, perhaps you should choose a small dog that can travel with you in the plane cabin. Your loyal dog will be unhappy without you or you will have greatly increased expenses, because you will have to hire a dog sitter or leave them in a kennel.

Another crime that only CSI could solve.

Allergies – Do I prefer a very tidy house? Do I have allergies? Many breeds constantly shed their hair, which means that there are better choices for allergy sufferers and neat freaks.

Time – Does my family take up all my spare time and are my children old enough to handle a puppy? A dog is like a child that never grows up and in order for them to be happy and well-behaved family members, they require a lot of your daily time and attention.

Fitness – Am I physically fit and healthy enough to be out there walking a dog two to three times a day, every day, rain or shine, and much more during the puppy stage? Do I have the time to involve them in a canine sport or job?

Cost – Am I able to afford the extra food costs, trips to the grooming parlour, health insurance, licensing, appropriate clothing and the veterinarian expenses that are part of being a conscientious Dachshund guardian?

Commitment – Is the decision to bring a puppy or dog into my life a family decision, or just because the children, who may quickly lose interest, have been begging for a dog?

Why? – What is the number one reason why I want a dog in my life?

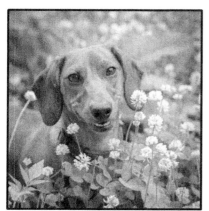

Once you ask yourself these important questions and honestly answer them, you will have gained a much better understanding of whether or not you have what it takes to share your life with a dog, and perhaps the beginning insight of the type of puppy or dog that would be best suited for you and your family.

If you're too busy for a dog, or choose the wrong dog that is not compatible with you or your family's energy and lifestyle (or you don't really have the time, finances, patience, expertise and commitment necessary to properly socialize, train, exercise, feed, raise and care for a canine companion), you will inevitably end up with an unhappy dog, which will lead to behavioral issues, which then will lead to a stressed family, angry neighbors, and in a best case scenario, extra expenses to hire a professional to help you reverse unwanted behavioral problems.

Even worse, an incompatible choice can mean that you may end up contributing to the already overflowing crisis of yet another dog being abandoned at the local SPCA or kill shelter.

Once you have done all your homework, and absolutely determined that the loyal, little Dachshund is the right dog for you (see next Section: The Ideal Guardian), rather than simply leaving it to chance, you need to choose the right puppy from the litter.

Generally speaking, when choosing a puppy out of a litter, look for one that is friendly and outgoing, rather than one who is overly aggressive or fearful.

Visit the breeder and take note of a puppy's social skills when they are still with their littermates, because this will help you to choose the right puppy for your family. Puppies who demonstrate good social skills with their littermates are much more likely to develop into easy-going, happy adults who play well with other dogs.

In a social setting where all the puppies can be observed together, there are several important observations you can make, including:

Play – Notice which puppies are comfortable both on top and on the bottom when play fighting and wresting with their littermates, and which puppies seem to only like being on top. Puppies who don't mind being on the bottom or who appear to be fine with either position will usually play well with other dogs when they become adults.

Sharing – Observe which puppies try to keep the toys away from the other puppies and which puppies share. Those who want to hoard the toys and keep all other puppies away may be more aggressive with other dogs over food or treats, or in play where toys are involved as they become older.

Company – Notice which puppies seem to like the company of the other pups and which ones seem to be loners. Puppies who like the company of their littermates are more likely to be interested in the company of other dogs as they mature than anti-social puppies.

Compassion – Observe the reaction of puppies that get yelped at when they bite or roughhouse with another puppy too hard. Puppies who ease up when another puppy yelps or cries are more likely to respond appropriately when they play too roughly as adults.

Sociability – Check to see if the puppy you are interested in is sociable with people, because if they will not come to you, or display fear of strangers, this may develop into a fear/aggression problem when they become adults.

Handling – Check if the puppy you are interested in is relaxed about being handled, because if they are not, they may become difficult or overly nervous around adults and children during daily interactions, during grooming or while visiting the veterinarian's office.

Is Your Happy Puppy Healthy?

While mental health is very important, you will also want to do all you can to determine if your chosen puppy is physically healthy.

First, ask to see veterinarian reports from the breeder to satisfy yourself that the puppy is as healthy as possible, and then once you make your decision to share your life with a particular puppy, and they are old enough to bring home, make an appointment with your own veterinarian for a complete examination.

However, before you take your new puppy home, there are general signs of good health to be aware of, including the following:

Body Fat – a healthy puppy will look round and well fed, with an obvious layer of fat over their rib cage.

Breathing – a healthy puppy will breathe quietly, without coughing, wheezing or sneezing.

Coat Condition – a healthy puppy will not be itchy and will have a soft coat with no dandruff, dullness, greasiness or bald spots.

Energy Level – a well-rested puppy will be alert and energetic.

Hearing – a healthy puppy should react if you clap your hands or snap your fingers behind their head.

Genitals – a healthy puppy will not have any sort of discharge visible in or around their genital or anal regions.

Mobility – a healthy puppy will walk and run normally without wobbling, limping or seeming to be weak, stiff or sore.

Vision – a healthy puppy will have bright, clear eyes without crust or discharge and they should notice if a ball is rolled past or a toy is tossed within their field of vision.

The Ideal Guardian

Once you have established that you have what it takes to share your life with a dog (by considering the questions in the previous Section), you should consider the following tips to determine whether the Dachshund would be the right breed for you and your family.

The Dachshund will be an excellent choice for moderate to high-energy individuals or families with older children that understand how to respect a dog that needs his or her own space. This dog can also be a good companion for senior adults who have the energy, time and mobility required to provide this companion (that always wants to be with you) with the daily exercise and mental stimulation they need.

Keep in mind that while a well-socialized Dachshund will usually be accepting of both unknown dogs and humans, when not trained to heed their guardian's lead, this feisty companion can easily become an unstable, stubborn, barking nightmare. Any dog that is babied too much can develop behavior problems. For instance, it is definitely possible for this small hound dog to become snappish if they think leadership has defaulted to them.

The ideal guardian for the Happy Dachshund will be a person who understands the importance of firms rules and boundaries for their dog, who is retired or works at home, and enjoys several moderate to high energy daily walks and some time for play. Also, for those more energetic dogs, a canine sport would be fun for everyone. This guardian will also be aware of this dog's strong desire to always be in close quarters with their favorite human, and that they may develop depression and separation anxiety if they are expected to spend long hours alone every day.

This ideal guardian will also understand the basics of socializing and gentle, fair training, without raised voices, and depending on the energy level of a particular dog, may also enjoy teaching this companion a fun canine sport, and be willing to involve him or her in their own daily walking or hiking routine.

As an example, the ideal happy Dachshund guardian will be someone who works at home or is retired, and takes his or her dog out for a 20 or 30 minute walk, so they can empty their bladder and bowels first thing every morning before breakfast, rain or shine.

After returning home, everyone will have their breakfast and then (since you work at home or are retired) your dog can relax on the couch for a couple of hours while you work about the home. Before long it's noon and time to leash up your little shadow companion and head off for another walk. Depending on the weather, you may finish up at a securely fenced local dog park for some socializing or play with other small dogs. If it's a hot day out, always carry water for your dog, and don't let them play too long.

Back home for a midday dental snack for your dog and lunch for you, while you take time (depending on this dog's age) to teach basic commands, play a short game, or maybe teach some tricks before your dog has a snooze and you get back to your time at home.

Now it's about 4:00 pm and again it's time to get you and your dog outside for a 20-30 minute walk, and if it's not too hot or too cold out, perhaps another short stop at the park. Keep in mind that if you live where the winters are harsh and you have access to a treadmill, this little dog can quickly be taught to exercise indoors alongside you on a treadmill.

TIP *Cold or wet weather will mean that this small dog needs a raincoat or a warm winter coat when walking outside. The Dachshund is not a fan of wet or cold weather and they may refuse to go outside.*

Don't give in, because they must still go outside to relieve themselves, even if it's just for a shortened time (unless you have trained them to use an indoor bathroom).

Back home and time to prepare dinner for both dog and human, then after dinner (again depending on the age of your dog) perhaps a few more minutes of basic command and/or trick training before you each have some lazy time in front of the fire or TV screen.

Now it's getting to be later evening and before bed you need to put your Dachshund on leash and take them outside for a few minutes so they can drain out their bladder before bed.

Everyone now in his or her respective beds as both human and dog have a rejuvenating sleep before the start of the next day when you do this (or something similar) all over again.

Of course, this is just one scenario that would be excellent for the Happy Dachshund, and with a little imagination on your part, there are many others that would fit the bill quite nicely.

Also, don't forget to check out your local weekend canine sporting facilities, and take the time to get you and your dog involved, because your weekend would be well spent teaching this dog how to run an Agility course, or perhaps participate in Advanced Obedience, Barn Hunt or even a Trick Training competition.

In a Nutshell

While learning how to choose the right puppy is important, even more important is your ability to ask and honestly answer the questions outlined in this Chapter that will help you to understand if you truly are a good fit for being the ideal guardian for the loyal and loving Dachshund, who will be your devoted companion.

Remember that if you don't really have the time, commitment and knowledge necessary to properly socialize and raise this fearless, short-legged companion, you will inevitably end up with an unhappy dog, which will lead to health and behavioral issues, which then will lead to a stressed family, possibly angry neighbors, and extra expenses to hire a professional to help you reverse unwanted behavioral problems.

Chapter 10: Humans Make a LOT of Stupid Mistakes

"Heaven goes by favor. If it went by merit, you would stay out and your dog would go in."
— Mark Twain

Far too often we humans don't even realize we are the cause of creating behavioral problems in our canine companions, and when we're not aware and paying attention, we may be causing a lot of issues that can actually be entirely avoided.

Besides the more obvious problems that can arise with a dog that is bred for tracking, hunting, search and rescue or detection work and can become a unhappy member of your family when not raised properly and engaged in a working capacity, there are many other situations or unwanted outcomes that may arise that can be avoided.

For instance, there are plenty of mistakes we humans can make, without even realizing it, that can send the wrong messages to our dogs, including:

🐾 not taking the time to properly socialize

- 🐾 forgetting about desensitizing to loud noises

- 🐾 falling prey to those pleading eyes

- 🐾 allowing a cute puppy to do something that will not be so cute once they have grown into an adult

- 🐾 feeding or treating too much

- 🐾 not exercising enough

- 🐾 not immediately correcting bad behavior

- 🐾 picking them up at the wrong time

- 🐾 rewarding them at the wrong time

- 🐾 bribing with treats, instead of teaching trust & respect

- 🐾 not being a strong enough leader

- 🐾 allowing him or her to be the boss

- 🐾 not taking the time to teach basic rules and boundaries

All of these and more can soon lead to plenty of trouble in later life and create unhappiness and unwanted behavior and health issues that could have been avoided.

As well, not being aware of the adolescent craziness time in a young dog's life and how to get through it, and many other less obvious mistakes, such as choosing the wrong collar or leash, sleeping in your bed, or free feeding can all result in the creation of problems.

While we humans may be well meaning, besides the obvious disasters that we can create when we don't properly train or socialize our canine friends, we can inadvertently make a lot of stupid mistakes when raising our canine companions that will cause our fur friends to needlessly suffer.

Let's begin with the more obvious *"Preventing Socialization Behavioral Issues"* that can lead to problems later in life, and proceed further into areas of *"Accidental Rewards"* that may not be so obvious, then touch upon *"Basic Rules and Boundaries"* and *"Adolescent Craziness"*, and finish this chapter with *"Less Obvious Stupid Human Mistakes"*.

Preventing Socialization Behavioral Issues

In order to prevent behavioral issues you first need to be aware of how easy it is to inadvertently create them yourself.

Much of how your Dachshund learns to behave will depend entirely upon you, how extensively they were socialized as a puppy and how much they are continually being socialized throughout their life.

Without proper socialization, even the most naturally friendly dog can become neurotic, unsociable and learn to act out aggressively toward unknown dogs, smaller animals or people. This is a situation that can get a small dog labelled nasty or even dangerous should they act out aggressively for any reason.

Many people don't realize how important it is to properly and continually socialize their dogs, even smaller ones like the Dachshund, in several different areas.

 Without proper socialization, many behavioral problems could easily become a daily occurrence.

Never make the mistake of thinking that you only need to socialize your Dachshund puppy during the first few months of their life and that they will then be fine for the rest of their life, because all dogs require constant socializing.

As well, once they reach adolescence, their personality can really begin to assert itself, and this is when, without constant and vigilant daily socializing and training, any aggressive or anti-social tendencies may begin to erupt.

Generally speaking, the majority of an adult dog's habits and behavioral traits will be formed between the ages of birth and one year of age. While it is even more important to introduce puppies to a wide variety of sights, sounds, smells and situations during the most formative period in their young life, which is usually their first 16 weeks, all dogs, no matter their age, need to be exposed to different people, dogs, animals, places and unusual sights and sounds throughout their entire adult life.

Socializing With Unknown Dogs

Any dog, despite their natural personality, that is not regularly socialized may become shy, nervous, afraid or suspicious around unfamiliar or unusual dogs, animals, people or circumstances, which could lead to nervous or fearful behavior, which can then lead to unacceptable aggression.

Daily on-leash dog walks are great opportunities for your Dachshund to see and possibly meet other dogs and different people, as well as practice proper behavior when out and about.

Remember to take it slowly and never put your dog in a situation where he or she feels uncomfortable or feels forced into being around other canines. Your dog should always be given the option to walk away, with lots of space.

When socializing a young puppy, remember to introduce him or her first to the *more calm and friendlier* of dogs, because introducing your tiny pup to a dog that may be overly boisterous or not so friendly with other dogs may result in a negative experience. Also keep in mind that many adult dogs simply don't have the patience for rambunctious puppies that eagerly invade another's space, and have not yet learned proper greeting etiquette.

Negative experiences at a young age may later result in a fear of other dogs. I would suggest finding a local puppy class with around 8-10 other puppies, so that you can carefully supervise socializing and guided play.

Socializing With Unknown People

Proper socialization also means taking your puppy (or dog) everywhere with you and introducing them to many different people of all ages, sizes and ethnicities, so they will learn what is normal and acceptable in their daily life.

TIP *DO NOT get into the habit of always carrying this small puppy or dog. They need to walk on their own feet so that they don't develop unwanted behavior problems, such as "armpit alligator" tendencies (snapping when someone stops to say hello) that can result from being in an elevated position where the dog feels they are in charge and must protect their human.*

Also important, will be getting your puppy or dog used to the noise and unpredictable actions of young children. You will want to closely supervise play, so that children are not accidentally being too rough or screaming in high-pitched voices, because this can be very frightening for a sensitive young puppy or dog that is unfamiliar with children.

Be especially careful when introducing your puppy to young children who may accidentally hurt your puppy, because you don't want your dog to become

fearful of children as this could lead to aggression issues later on in life.

When this puppy gets a little older, they will not hesitate to bite a child that is invading their space or treating them roughly.

Environmental Socialization

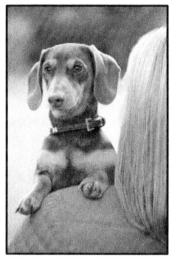

It can be a BIG mistake not to take the time to introduce your Dachshund puppy to a wide variety of different environments, because when they are not comfortable with different sights, smells and sounds, this could cause them (and you) stress and trauma later in their adult life.

Be creative and take your puppy everywhere you can imagine when they are young, so that no matter where they travel, whether strolling along a noisy city sidewalk or beside a peaceful shoreline, they will be equally comfortable. Also, don't forget to train a miniature Dachshund to like travelling inside their very useful Sherpa bag.

Do not make the mistake of only taking your puppy into areas where you live and will frequently travel, because they need to also be comfortable visiting areas you might not often visit, such as noisy construction sites, airports or a shopping area across town.

Your puppy needs to see all sorts of sights, sounds and situations so that they will not become fearful, should they need to travel with you outside of their immediate neighbourhood.

Your Dachshund will take their cues from you, which means that when you are calm and in control of every situation, they will learn to be the same because they will trust and calmly follow your lead.

For instance, take them to a noisy construction site, to the airport where they can watch people and hear planes landing and taking off, to a local park where they can see a baseball game, for a stroll beside a schoolyard at recess time when noisy children are out playing, or to the local zoo or farm and let them get a close up look at horses, pigs and ducks. Use your imagination.

Again, never think that socialization is something that only takes place when your Dachshund is a young puppy, as proper socialization is on-going for your dog's entire life.

Fear of Loud Noises

Many dogs can show extreme fear of loud noises, such as fireworks, sirens, thunderstorms or home security alarms. We humans need to learn how to either prevent this trauma in the first place or learn how to appropriately respond to a dog that is afraid of loud noises.

When you take the time to desensitize your dog to these types of noises when they are very young, it will be much easier on them during stormy weather, holidays such as Halloween or New Year's, when fireworks are often a part of the festivities, when an ambulance or fire truck roars past with sirens wailing, or when your fire or security alarm is activated.

REMEMBER: Dogs have superior hearing and loud, piercing noises will be very painful for them, so protect their ears if you're out walking when a vehicle with a blaring siren is roaring past.

Desensitization Devices: there are several ways you can help to desensitize your Dachshund, so that they are not fearful of high-pitched alarms, and loud, popping noises, including the following:

CDs: you can purchase CD's that are a collection of unusual sounds, such as vacuums or hoovers, airplanes, sirens, smoke alarms, fireworks, people clapping hands, screaming children, and more (or you can easily make your own), that you can play while working in your kitchen or relaxing in your living room or lounge.

When you play these sounds and pretend that everything is normal, the next time your puppy or dog hears these types of sounds elsewhere, they will not become upset or agitated because they have learned to ignore them.

Bubble Wrap: is also another simple way to desensitize a Dachshund that is fearful of unexpected sounds. Show them the bubble wrap, pop a few of the cells and if they do not run away, give them a treat. You can start with the bubble wrap that has small, quieter cells, and then graduate them to the larger celled (louder) bubble wrap. You can also take things even farther by blowing up some small paper bags or balloons and loudly popping them in front of your dog, or taking them to the rifle range.

Thunder Shirts: some dogs will respond well to wearing a *"Thunder Shirt"*, which is specifically designed to alleviate anxiety or trauma associated with loud rumbling, popping or banging noises. The idea behind the design of the Thunder Shirt is that the gentle pressure it creates is similar to a hug that, for some dogs, has a calming effect.

Relaxation Collars: there are basically two types of collars designed to help relax or calm an upset puppy or dog. One uses scent or calming pheromones, while the other uses species-specific music at appropriate decibel levels to calm a fearful or stressed dog.

TV or Radio: sometimes all that is required to calm a dog that is stressed by loud noises is to play your inside TV or Radio station with the sounds of relaxing music, louder than you might normally, to help disguise the exterior noise of fireworks or thunder.

Always be aware that some dogs literally lose their minds and do things that make no logical sense when they hear the loud popping or screeching noises of fireworks and various alarms and start trembling, running or trying to hide and you cannot communicate with them at all.

Make certain that your dog cannot harm itself trying to escape from these types of noises, and if possible, calmly hold them until they begin to relax.

For instance, my dog, Boris, used to try and escape through the drain in the bathtub (go figure), because loud popping noises literally caused him to lose his mind.

Make sure that YOU are acting appropriately yourself, by not panicking or having weak, *"feeling sorry"* or *"angry and frustrated"* energy around an upset dog, because this will only make matters worse.

When the person who is supposed to be your dog's support system is also feeling weak or acting unstable, your dog will have nowhere to turn. Instead, support them by pretending that nothing is wrong and if you must talk to them, do so in a calm, yet assertive voice.

Never underestimate the importance of taking the time to continually (not just when they are puppies) socialize and desensitize your Dachshund to all manner of sounds. Doing so will help curb their tendency to sound off at every little noise, which will make everyone happier in the future, while teaching them to be a calm and well-balanced member of your family in every situation.

Accidental Rewards

Many times, we humans are guilty of accidentally rewarding our puppies and dogs for engaging in types of behavior we are not happy with, and the following are some of the more obvious things we may be doing that are inadvertently rewarding, and thus encouraging, an unwanted behavior.

Aggression Rewards

Many people unknowingly get into the habit of accidentally rewarding their puppies or dogs for displaying nervousness, fear, barking, growling or lunging at another dog or person by picking them up, talking soothingly, or offering them a treat. I see this happen all too often.

For instance, many people with smaller dogs, like the Dachshund, simply pick up their dog when he or she is acting in an unacceptable manner. Do NOT get into this bad habit.

Should you accidentally reward your dog when they are displaying any sort of unbalanced energy, this actually turns out to be a reward for them, and you will be teaching them to continue with this type of unwanted behavior.

As well, picking up a small dog or puppy when they are growling, barking or acting out inappropriately, again rewards them and places them in a top dog position where they literally have just gained the higher ground.

A dog in the *"top dog"* position feels more confident and, depending on your energy, will usually then become more dominant than the person or dog they may have just growled at when they were at *"ground level"*.

Rather than accidentally rewarding your Dachshund for displaying unwanted behavior, the correct action to take in such a situation is to keep them on the ground, and gently correct your puppy or dog with firm yet calm energy (that is just a little stronger than the energy your dog is displaying) by distracting them with a firm *"No!"* and a quick sideways snap of the leash to get their attention back on you. This will "tell" your dog that they must let you deal with whatever situation has caused them to react badly.

If you allow a fearful, nervous or shy dog to deal with situations that unnerve them and cause them to bellow loudly or act out aggressively when they encounter unfamiliar circumstances, you will have created a problem that could escalate into something very serious.

The same is true of situations where a young puppy may feel the need to protect itself from a larger or older dog that may come charging in for a sniff or is acting confrontational. It's the human guardian's responsibility to protect their puppy or dog, so that they do not feel that they must react with fear or aggression in order to protect his or herself or the human at the other end of the leash.

 No matter the age or size of your Dachshund puppy or dog, allowing them to display aggression or any sort of unwanted behavior toward another dog, animal or person is NEVER a laughing matter and this type of behavior must be immediately curtailed.

Excitement Rewards

It's important to recognize that attention paid to an overly excited or out-of-control puppy or dog, even negative attention, is likely going to be rewarding for your fur friend. If your dog is not receiving enough of your attention, they will quickly learn to do whatever it takes to get the attention they desire.

Bottom line, when you engage with an out-of-control puppy or dog, you end up actually rewarding them for acting out in an unstable manner, and encouraging them to continue with more overly exuberant behavior you might not be very pleased about.

Be careful that you're not teaching your dog to act out with crazy energy every time they see you.

For instance, chasing after a puppy when they have taken something they are not supposed to have, picking them up when they are barking or showing aggression, pushing them off when they jump on you or other people, or yelling when they refuse to come when called, are all forms of attention that can actually be rewarding and encourage more of the same behavior.

Instead, remain calm and assertive and be consistent with your training, so that your dog learns how to control their energy and play quietly and appropriately without jumping on everyone or engaging in growling, barking or mouthy behavior.

Interaction Rewards

If your Dachshund displays excited energy simply from being petted by you, or anyone else, you will need to teach yourself, your family and your friends to ignore your fur friend until he or she calms down. Otherwise, you will be inadvertently teaching your canine companion that the touch of humans means excitement, and this behavioral problem will continue to escalate.

For instance, when you continue to engage with your overly excited puppy or dog, you are actually rewarding them for out-of-control behavior and literally teaching them that when they see humans, you want them to display excited energy.

Too many people encourage their dog to be nuts, for instance, when they return home and greet their dog in a highly excited state. While it's nice to know that your dog is happy to see you, when you forget about being your dog's calm pack leader just a few times, this may be enough to send your dog the message that they can no longer rely upon you to be their leader, and that seeing humans means they must now display out-of-control excitement.

Instead, when you come home, do what's best for your dog. Greet him or her calmly and quietly, and if they are at all excited, do NOT touch or talk to them until they calm down. Otherwise, your leadership will have vanished and your dog will soon learn that humans are a source of excitement. Once this has happened, long, consistently vigilant work on your part (with help from your friends and family) will be the only way to reverse this unwanted behavior.

Another thing to keep in mind is that children are often a source of high energy and excitement that can cause a puppy or dog to quickly become extremely wound up.

If you don't want to create an on-going behavioral problem, that could accidentally get someone injured, you will need to be very vigilant about NOT permitting young children to engage with an excited puppy or dog.

Important Basic Rules and Boundaries

You can prevent many future behavioral problems when you take the time to ensure that your Dachshund learns basic rules and boundaries. All that's necessary for effectively teaching your puppy (or dog) these basics is a calm, consistent and firm approach, combined with your endless patience.

Basic rules and boundaries would include things such as:

- 🐾 no barking at every little noise

- 🐾 no dogs allowed in the kitchen when preparing food

- 🐾 no begging at the human's dinner table

- 🐾 humans through the door first

- 🐾 no sleeping in the human bed

- 🐾 no raiding the garbage can

- 🐾 no jumping up on tables or counters

- 🐾 no helping yourself to "tootsie rolls" from the cat's litter box

- 🐾 no chasing the neighbor's cat

Many puppies are ready to begin basic training at about 10 to 12 weeks of age, and some will be ready at 8 weeks. However, be careful not to overdo it when they are less than four months of age, as their attention span may be short.

With younger puppies, make your training sessions no more than 5 or 10 minutes, positive and pleasant with plenty of praise and/or treats, so that your puppy will be looking forward to their next session.

Also, begin to introduce hand signals that go along with the verbal commands so that once they learn both, you can remove the verbal commands in favor of just hand signals.

Consistently teach your puppy or dog the *All Important Three*, which is the "Come", "Sit" and "Stay" commands (more about this in Chapter 12: Training Basics For a Happy Dachshund), and use them every day in every opportunity to help your young dog progress through their unpredictable adolescent period.

Adolescent Craziness

Too often, we humans become impatient and frustrated and give up on our dogs when they transition from being the cute, cuddly and mostly obedient little puppy they once were and become all kinds of craziness.

Instead of riding the adolescent storm, it is often during this confusing and trying adolescent stage of a dog's life that they end up behind bars when the humans who promised to love and protect them, abandon their once happy fur friend at the local SPCA or rescue facility.

With consistency, understanding, the right information, and endless patience and perseverance, you and your fur friend can emerge out the other side of this adolescent period with a much stronger bond.

Firstly, you need to know that not all dogs go through an intensely crazy adolescent period. Secondly, when you remain consistent with your socializing and training during this time, you can live through puppy adolescence and come out the other side a much more knowledgeable and patient guardian.

Remember, you've already lived through potty training, teething, socializing and basic rules and boundaries with your young Dachshund, and you need to feel proud of all your accomplishments and the leaps and bounds you and your puppy have accomplished together over the last several months.

If your adolescent dog is now beginning to act out and push your buttons, rather than giving up on them, it's time to remain calm, consistent and persistent, and re-visit basic rules and boundaries, while keeping in mind that you will eventually be able to enjoy the happy rewards that all those months of diligent puppy training have brought to your relationship.

During adolescence, you may experience several changes in your dog's personality that you're not exactly pleased about. For instance, your young Dachshund may:

- 🐾 no longer be as friendly with strangers

- 🐾 start to be possessive of their human

- 🐾 begin to be possessive of their food and toys

- 🐾 start to bark at unknown people and dogs

- 🐾 think the neighbor's cat is fair game

- 🐾 show their teeth when someone invades their space

- 🐾 start to show their stubborn side

- 🐾 ignore you when called

- 🐾 dig up the back yard

- 🐾 appear to have suddenly gone deaf

- 🐾 ignore the basic commands they've already learned

- 🐾 start to relieve themselves inside again

- 🐾 bark or howl when left alone

- 🐾 begin to mark territory

- 🐾 refuse to go walking in the rain

Welcome to the world of canine adolescence, where it appears that all your previous work was for naught and your puppy has turned into some sort of uncontrollable monster.

DON'T PANIC, because every dog is different and your dog's adolescent period may go by without notice. However, being prepared for the worst will help you ride any impending storm and get you both safely out the other side where you can enjoy an even closer relationship than you previously had.

The adolescent phase may be very subtle for your puppy or on the other hand, it may be so dramatic that frustration with your fur friend is becoming a daily occurrence.

If frustration is getting the upper hand, rather than letting it get worse, consider the benefits of hiring a professional, who can provide insight and valuable assistance to help you through this stage of your puppy's development.

Less Obvious Stupid Human Mistakes

There are many less obvious mistakes we humans can inadvertently make with our dogs that can also lead to behavioral problems later in life, some of which include:

Sleeping in Your Bed: many people make the mistake of allowing a crying puppy to sleep with them in their bed. While this may help to calm and comfort a new puppy, it will set a dangerous precedent that can result in behavioral problems later in their life, plus a sleeping human body could easily crush a tiny Dachshund puppy.

As much as it may pull on your heart strings to hear your new puppy crying the first couple of nights in their kennel, a little tough love at the beginning will keep them safe while helping them to learn to both love and respect you as their leader.

Picking Them Up at the Wrong Time: never pick your puppy up if they display nervousness, fear or aggression (such as growling or barking) toward an object, person or other pet, because this will be rewarding them for unbalanced behavior.

Instead, your puppy needs to be gently corrected by you, with firm and calm energy, so that they learn not to react with fear or aggression.

Armpit Alligators: when your Dachshund is a small size, be aware that many guardians get into the bad habit of carrying a small dog or puppy far too much.

Remember that they need to be on the ground and walking on their own, so that they do not become overly confident. A dog that is carried by their guardian is literally being placed in the *"top dog"* position.

Be aware that humans who constantly carry small dogs or puppies, rather than allowing them to walk on their own, can often inadvertently create what I refer to as an *"armpit alligator"* situation. This is where you see someone carrying a cute little dog and you stop to say hello, only to be greeted by snapping jaws and sharp teeth.

Even dogs that are friendly and not naturally wary or suspicious of strangers can learn to become intolerant if they don't receive adequate socialization, which means that it is always possible to allow them to become protective or possessive of *"their"* humans.

Playing Too Hard or Too Long: many humans play too hard or allow their children to play too long or too roughly with their puppy. You need to remember that your young puppy tires very easily and especially during the critical growing phases of their young life, they need their rest.

Hand Play: always discourage your puppy from chewing or biting your hands, or any part of your body for that matter.

Do NOT get into the habit of playing the *"hand"* game, where you rough up your puppy and slide them across the floor with your hands, because this will teach them that your hands are playthings and you will have to work hard to break this bad habit.

PERSONAL EXPERIENCE: When my puppy came home with me at 10-weeks of age, the breeder had already been playing the hand game and it took me a very long time to teach my Boris that biting human hands was not acceptable behavior. Interestingly, when he sees people that he has not seen for years, that he used to know when he was a young puppy, this old habit often re-surfaces for a short while.

When your puppy is teething, they will naturally want to chew on everything within reach, and this will include you. As cute as you might think it is, this is not an acceptable behavior and you need to gently, but firmly, discourage the habit.

A light flick with a finger on the end of your puppy's nose, combined with a firm "NO" and removing the enticing fingers by making a fist when they are trying to bite human fingers, will discourage them from this activity.

Not Getting Used to Grooming: not taking the time to get your Dachshund used to a regular grooming routine, including bathing, brushing, toenail clipping and teeth brushing, can lead to a lifetime of trauma for both human and dog every time these procedures must be performed.

 Set aside a few minutes each day for your grooming routine.

NOTE: Get your puppy used to being up high on a table or countertop when you are grooming them. This way, when it comes time for a full grooming session or a visit to the vet's office, where they will be placed on an examination table, they will not be stressed because this will already be a familiar situation.

Free Feeding: means to keep food in your puppy's bowl 24/7, so that they can eat any time of the day or night, whenever they feel like it.

While free feeding a young puppy can be a good idea (especially with very small dogs), until they are about four or five months old, many guardians often get into the bad habit of allowing their adult dogs to continue to eat food any time they want, by leaving food out 24/7.

The Dachshund may be quite food motivated, and can quickly become overweight if you feed too much. However, every dog is different, and it's never a good idea to get into the habit of leaving food out 24/7 because (a) they no longer associate you being in control of the food, and (b) if your particular dog gets used to eating too much, they will quickly gain weight and become obese.

Getting into a free feeding habit can be a serious mistake, as your dog is not a cat, and needs to know that you are absolutely in control of their food.

Treating Them Like Children: do not get into the bad habit of treating your dog like a small, furry human; even though they may try their best to please you and their doggy smarts could help them to succeed in most instances, not honoring them for being the amazing dog they are will only cause them confusion that could lead to behavioral problems.

 Remember that the one thing your dog is the absolute BEST at, is Being a Dog.

A well-balanced dog thrives on rules and boundaries, and when they understand that there is no question that you are their leader and they are your follower, they will live a contented, happy and stress-free life.

Distraction and Replacement: when your puppy tries to chew on your hand, foot, clothing, or anything else that is not fair game, you need to firmly and calmly tell them "No", and then distract them by replacing what they are not supposed to be chewing with something they <u>are</u> permitted to chew, such as an appropriate toy.

Make sure that you happily praise them every time they choose the toy to chew on. If your puppy persists in chewing on you, remove yourself from the equation by getting up and walking away. If they are really persistent, put them inside their kennel with a favorite chew toy until they calm down.

Always praise your puppy when they stop inappropriate behavior or replace inappropriate behavior with something that is acceptable to you, so that they begin to understand what they can and cannot do.

Flat Collar Nightmares

Many humans simply don't realize how important it is to choose the "right" kind of collar for their canine companion. Add this to the fact that there is an ever-increasing array of tempting colors and styles to choose from and it's very easy to get distracted and forget about choosing what you really need for your dog.

What you really need in a collar is one that will also keep your Dachshund safe and secure. While the flat collar may be fine for a calm dog that never pulls, leaps about or suddenly tries to do an about face and take off running in a different direction to chase that teasing squirrel or taunting cat, this is not a very safe reality.

While you will choose what you will for your dog, after 40 some years of working with dogs and experiencing possibly every type of terrifying, unexpected disaster while out walking a dog, the ONLY collar I feel absolutely confident using (because I know that the dog I'm in control of cannot wiggle out of it), is the "Martingale" collar.

Flat collars, unless you have them cinched up so tight that you're almost cutting off your dog's air supply, can be fairly easy for most dogs to get out of.

All dogs are amazing athletes, and even though you may have a firm grip on that leash, they can back away from you, wiggle, twist and contort themselves in a quick instant, flip their head and the collar is off – bye, bye doggy!

The Martingale Collar

There are several reasons why the Martingale dog collar is far superior to a flat collar:

- 🐾 comfortable for your dog to wear

- 🐾 safe because your dog cannot wiggle out of it

- 🐾 best training collar

The Martingale collar looks much the same as a flat collar, with one very important difference – there is a triangular piece of chain in the middle of it. This chain is attached to the collar with two rings, with a third ring in the middle of the chain, which is where you attach your leash.

When there is no tension on the collar (from them pulling on the leash), the collar hangs loose and comfortable. However, when there IS tension on the collar, that little piece of chain tightens so that your dog cannot get out of their collar.

PERSONAL EXPERIENCE: My dog (despite his short nose) has been wearing the same Martingale "training" collar for over 14 years and will continue to do so, because this collar conveys important messages between my dog and myself.

That little piece of triangular chain makes a slight noise when you sharply tug or jiggle it, and this sends a message to your dog that you want their attention on you. It's simply the best collar for teaching your dog to walk calmly by your side and to remind them that YOU are in charge.

When buying a Martingale collar for your Dachshund, take him or her with you because it needs to be the correct size to fit over the widest part of their head. Then, once you've got the right size for your dog, you need to pay strict attention to the <u>correct way to</u> <u>adjust</u> the collar for maximum effect and safety.

Adjusting the Martingale Collar: once you've placed the collar over your dog's head, you need to adjust the length so that when you attach the leash to the outside ring and pull it tight, when the two inside rings come together, there is still a gap between these two rings of approximately two human finger widths. You never want the two inside rings to touch.

You can now enjoy comfortable and safe walks with your Happy Dachshund companion.

<u>Flexi-Leash Fiasco</u>

Personally, flexi, retractable or extendable dog leashes are high on my list of pet peeves, for several important reasons, because they:

- ❧ are dangerous for human and dog alike

- ❧ allow the dog to be in the wrong walking position

- ❧ allow the humans to forget their responsibilities

- ❧ are difficult to securely grip

- ❧ are an excuse for not properly training your dog

- ❧ can accidentally break

While many people believe that a retractable leash is a good way to allow their dogs more freedom to roam while still keeping them securely attached, the above reasons highlight why these leashes can be a very bad idea. See below for more details.

Injury to human and dog: these leashes are usually spring-loaded, many feet long (usually 26 feet or 7.9 meters), and thin cords wound up inside a cumbersome plastic compartment with a handle and a button to control how much of the leash is extended.

As you can imagine, it's far more difficult to control a dog that is roaming about 20 or more feet away from you, than it would be if they were attached to a standard 4 to 6 foot leash.

If your dog gets used to having a 20-foot (6 meter) or more leeway, they will be busy sniffing interesting scents, and can quickly run out into traffic, be surprised by another dog rushing in, or get tangled up with a person and a dog, which can cause both injury to the dogs and people, or may cause a fight between the two dogs.

These leashes are also serious tripping hazards that can cause many injuries.

MEMORY LANE: The daughter of one of my dog whispering clients broke her toe as a result of tripping over a flexi-leash, I have suffered painful "rope" burns several times, and once was hit in the head (ouch!) with the hard and heavy plastic handle as it snapped back when the person holding it lost their grip and dropped it.

In addition, every flexi or retractable leash is equipped with a brake to stop the unwinding of the cord at various lengths. If your dog is running and all of a sudden comes to the end of their freedom, unless you drop the handle, they will be forced to come to a very abrupt stop that can injure a dog's neck or spine.

Incorrect Walking Position: the ONLY place your dog should ever be when you're out walking is beside you, and when you allow them to freely roam 20 or more feet from wherever you are, besides being lax about teaching your dog the correct walking position, you are *"telling"* them that you are no longer in charge. A dog that believes they are in charge can get you BOTH into a lot of trouble.

Forgetting Your Human Responsibilities: when you're out walking with your puppy or dog, as their leader, you are responsible for everything they do, including picking up after them. A retractable leash allows your dog to literally be out of your sight. While you're busy chatting with a neighbor or checking your phone messages, who knows what sort of *"message"* your dog may be depositing in the neighbor's yard.

You can be fined for not picking up after your dog, not to mention gaining yourself a bad reputation from your neighbors or other more responsible dog walkers.

Difficult to Securely Grip: the flexi leash has a large, cumbersome handle that is quite slippery and difficult to securely hold onto. If your companion suddenly lunges or changes direction, the chances of you losing your grip are quite high, and when that happens, the consequences can be dangerously grave.

Once dropped, your dog is now dragging a bouncing, loudly clattering handle, which can be very noisy on a sidewalk or hard surface.

MEMORY LANE: This very thing has happened to me in a busy, high traffic area, when walking someone else's dog, and I can tell you from first-hand experience that this is a highly stressful and frightening situation I would not want to wish on anyone.

Unless your dog has been trained to remain calmly sitting while rifles are fired near their head, this flexi leash that seems to be chasing them can be a very scary experience that will cause most dogs to run.

When your dog is scared, they will run even faster, while you run after them adding to the chaos with your panic-stricken screams to stop before they get killed trying to cross a busy intersection. Not a good scene.

Poor Training: while many might believe they are giving their dog more freedom by using a retractable leash, they are actually missing out on properly training their dog to heel beside them and to respond appropriately to the all-important "come" or "recall" command.

The very nature of a flexi leash is such that the dog is often out in front of the person who is supposed to be in charge, and always *"pulling"*, which to an approaching dog can look like an aggressive stance, resulting in the other dog thinking he or she must retaliate with a defensive stance. All of this, as you can imagine, has the potential to result in a scuffle between dogs and humans.

Accidental Breakage: there is a great deal of wear on a small diameter cord that is constantly unwinding and rewinding and you may not notice a worn area until it actually breaks. Then, you've got a potential runaway dog disaster to hopefully recover from, before the dog gets severely injured or killed by a vehicle, or finds his or herself in some other type of serious trouble.

Improve your training, have better control, make your life easier, avoid injuries, and ensure the safety and security of yourself and your furry best friend by choosing a Martingale collar and a standard 4-foot leash.

Sled Dog Fiasco

One last thought about what I call the *"Sled Dog Fiasco"*. Many people think that buying a harness is a better choice than the proper collar for their canine companion. However, the only time a harness is actually the right choice is if you have a strong sled dog that you need to put in harness, so that they can pull you.

What happens when you put most dogs in a harness is that (1) they are automatically in the wrong walking position, being head and shoulders in front of you; (2) you no longer have control of their head and cannot correct unwanted behavior; and (3) they now are in control of you and are much more powerful and potentially difficult to control, because the entire weight and strength of their body is attached to that harness.

Take Away Tip: "Harnesses are for sled dogs".

In a Nutshell

It cannot be emphasized strongly enough how important it is to properly socialize your Dachshund puppy, and understand that we humans often unknowingly reward our dogs at the wrong time, which can actually cause behavioral issues later in life.

Re-visit this Chapter information and think about what other mistakes you may be inadvertently making, so that you can do your best to avoid simple mistakes we humans often are guilty of making with our dogs, that can lead to an unhappy dog that suffers from behavioral problems later in life.

Also, when training your puppy or dog, keep in mind that the type of leash and collar you choose can make a big difference.

Chapter 11: Happy Dachshund Body Language

*"Money can buy a fine dog, but
only love can make him wag his tail."*
— Kinky Friedman

We all know good communication is not just about the words we use. Our tone of voice, energy and our body language help to package up and deliver our meaning every day. While most people can effectively communicate their thoughts and feelings through words, we need to generally be reliant upon reading our dog's body language in order to know if they are happy or sad.

Because our dogs don't speak our language, the only way to truly comprehend and communicate with them is for us to understand and appreciate what they are telling us through their body and vocal language.

Often, gestures or actions that we assume mean one thing are actually the dog telling us the exact opposite, and determining what that wagging tail or barking really means can sometimes be the difference between a belly rub and a bite.

How happy would you be if you could not communicate with your family at home? Would you develop behaviour issues over time? Of course you would, and the same is also true for your beloved dog.

They need you to understand what they are "telling you" and how they feel, in order to be a happy family member. For instance, learning to properly "read" your dog's intentions can easily prevent an unwanted encounter during a visit to the local park.

Therefore, taking the time to educate yourself about basic canine body language and paying attention to your dog's body language (including their face, posture, barking and tail position) is an important prerequisite for raising a content and well-behaved dog.

This Chapter will teach you exactly that – to understand the basics of what your furry friend (and those dogs around you) are trying to "tell" you and how they feel, so that you can share a happy lifelong partnership together.

So, don't wait and read on.

What's With All the Wagging and Barking?

While a well-socialized Dachshund may often happily wag their tail, it can be a mistake to automatically assume that if your dog, or someone else's dog, is wagging their tail, they are happy and friendly.

What Does the Wag Mean?

When determining a dog's true intent or demeanor, it's important to take into consideration the complete dog posture, rather than just the tail, because it's entirely possible that a dog can be wagging his or her tail just before it decides to take an aggressive lunge toward you or your dog.

More important in determining the emotional state of most dogs is the height or positioning of their tail. For instance, a tail that is held parallel to your dog's back usually suggests that they are feeling relaxed, whereas if the tail is held stiffly vertical, this usually means that they may be feeling aggressive or dominant.

Also keep in mind that certain dog tails are carried differently for different reasons. Depending on which dog tail, you will have more or less visible cues. The opposite is also true of other dogs reading your dog's body language. For instance, a dog with a docked or tightly curled tail can sometimes send confusing messages to others.

A tail held much lower can mean that your dog is feeling stressed, afraid, submissive or unwell and if the tail is tucked underneath the dog's body, this is most often a sign that the dog is feeling highly stressed, nervous, fearful or threatened by another dog or person.

Paying attention to your dog's tail (and any dog tails around you) can help you to know when you need to step in and make some space between your dog and another, more dominant dog.

Of course, different breeds naturally carry their tails at different heights, some dogs have tightly curled tails and some dogs don't have any visible tails. So, you will need to take this into consideration so that you get used to their particular body language signals.

As well, the speed at which the tail is moving will give you an idea of the mental state of your dog, because the speed of the wag usually indicates how excited a dog may be.

For instance, a slow, slightly swinging wag can often mean that a dog is tentative about greeting another dog, and this is more of a questioning type of wag, whereas a fast-moving tail held high can mean that your dog is about to challenge or threaten another less dominant dog.

Also, a stalking stance, where your dog has raised hackles (hair along the back), lowers their head and slowly creeps forward with an intense stare often happens just before a serious attack. There is also a similar-looking *"play"* stance, and without practice, you may have difficulty identifying the difference between the two.

MEMORY LANE: I've been sworn at after politely letting a guardian of a larger dog, who was unaware (and didn't want to know) that their dog was stalking my smaller dog and about to do him harm, so be careful how you approach these situations.

What Does the Bark Mean?

Of course, our dogs bark for a wide variety of reasons, and every dog is different, depending upon their natural breed tendencies and how they were raised. Even though the Dachshund has the reputation for being a tenacious barker, when you take the time, you can certainly teach them not to bark unless absolutely necessary. This section discusses some of the more common reasons why a dog might be barking.

Communication: since the very first dog, they have communicated over long distances by howling to one another and when in closer proximity, barking to warn off other dogs approaching what they consider to be their territory, or in excitement or happiness when greeting another member of the dog pack.

Now, our domesticated dogs have learned to bark for a wide variety of reasons, such as when they sense danger or are alerting us to someone approaching the home. A dog will also bark in anticipation of their favorite food, when they are afraid, frustrated, bored, excited, or to let us know they want to play. Barking is an effective way to get the attention of us humans because barking is a loud and difficult noise to ignore.

Danger: many dogs will bark to alert us to visitors or intruders, and we need to learn how to understand the difference between what our dogs perceive as danger and what is truly dangerous, or indeed how to teach our best friends the difference.

We want our dogs to tell us when there is real, imminent danger and in this case, should the danger involve an unwanted intruder, we want them to bark loudly to possibly scare this threat away.

When our dogs are barking for a reason we are not yet aware of, we need to calmly assess the situation rather than immediately becoming annoyed.

We also need to remember that a Dachshund's sense of smell, hearing and sometimes eyesight is far more acute than our own, which means that we need to give them an opportunity to tell us if they just heard, saw or sensed something that they are worried or uncertain about.

Rather than ignoring our dogs (or yelling at them) when they are attempting to *"tell"* us that something is bothering them, even if we ourselves understand that the noise the dog just heard is only the neighbor's kids coming home from school or a postal delivery, we need to respond appropriately.

We need to <u>calmly</u> acknowledge our dog's concern by saying, *"OK, good dog,"* and then ask them to come to you. This way you have quietly and calmly let your dog know that the situation is nothing to be concerned about and you have asked them to move away from the target they are concerned about, which places you in control, and which will usually stop the barking.

Attention: many dogs will learn to bark to get their owner's attention, just because they are bored or want to be taken outside for an interesting walk or a trip to the local park to chase a ball.

Our canine companions are very good at manipulating us in this way, and if we fall for it, we are setting up an annoying precedent that could plague us for the remainder of our relationship.

MEMORY LANE: I shared my life with a Blue Heeler who would go berserk with loud barking every time we drove near a park or when we arrived at a park. Even so, I would never reward him for barking, because as annoying and hard on the eardrums as it was, I had to sit calmly inside the vehicle until he stopped barking. If I had let him immediately bound out of the vehicle, I would have inadvertently taught my dog that barking got him exactly what he wanted.

When a dog is barking to gain their guardian's attention, for whatever reason, before we immediately capitulate, first we need to calmly ask our dog to do something for us. After our dog has performed a calm and quiet task for us, such as sit or lie down, then we can decide to give our dog our undivided attention on our terms.

Often you will see a dog and their guardian at the local dog park playing fetch and when the human is not throwing that ball quickly enough to satisfy the dog's desire to run and fetch, the dog will be madly barking at the guardian. This is the equivalent of being sworn at in doggy language.

Don't make the mistake of allowing your puppy or dog to manipulate you in this situation, because if you do, you will soon create a bad habit that will very quickly become not just annoying to you, but also annoying to everyone else at the park.

Before throwing a ball or Frisbee for a dog that loves to retrieve, it's important to always ask the dog to sit and make eye contact with you.

Often the types of canines that are overly exuberant with chasing a ball or Frisbee (such as the Dachshund) have learned this barking behavior from their humans, who allowed themselves to be literally at the beck and call of their dog, and created this irritating habit by throwing the ball every time the dog barked.

In this situation, if you allow your dog to dictate to you when you will throw the ball, they will quickly learn that barking gets them their desired result, and you have just created an annoying, rude dog who is yelling at you in doggy language to do their bidding.

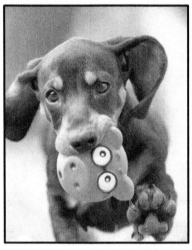

In this type of ball-retrieving scenario, the dog has become ball *"obsessed"* and is no longer really paying attention to the guardian's commands, as they are solely focusing on where the ball is.

While there are many situations in which your Dachshund may bark to convey that they've heard a noise, in all other situations where the barking is done to demand attention, a toy or an object or food, this is when you need to ask them to do something for you, and then only if you want to give them what they are asking for, do you follow through.

MEMORY LANE: I once had a client whose dog would start to loudly bark every time he answered the phone. This was big time annoying to everyone, and all of this could have been avoided if he had taken the time to properly train his dog to be respectful. The good news here is that once we completed a little dog whispering session and he became a stronger leader, the dog no longer barked when the phone rang.

Bottom line, remember to stay calm when your cute puppy is demanding attention, because even negative attention can be rewarding for your dog, and can lead down a future, unwanted path where he or she will learn further habits that will not be particularly endearing for the human side of the relationship when the cute puppy has become an adult.

Boredom or Separation Anxiety: many dogs, especially those who have not been properly trained, are treated like children, or that have not been allowed to understand that they have rules and boundaries, will sharply bark when left at home and are bored or are feeling the anxiety of being alone.

 Many times, we humans believe that our dog is barking when being left alone, because he or she is experiencing "separation anxiety", when in fact what the dog is really experiencing is the frustration of observing a member of the pack which they believe to be their follower (i.e. You) leaving them.

This can happen when you are not a strong enough leader for your loving, feisty and fearless little Dachshund and they have taken over. They may then loudly verbalize their frustration and displeasure because, in the dog world, the pack follower (which you have allowed yourself to be) does NOT leave the pack leader (them). *I've seen this type of situation many times over, and once the human side of the relationship steps up and takes control, it quickly reverses.*

Breaking your dog of the habit of loud barking when they are left alone can be solved in different ways, with the most obvious being that you simply take your dog with you wherever you go, because after all, they are pack animals, and in order for them to be really happy and well balanced, they need the constant direction of their leader (which is supposed to be you).

Another much more lengthy, time consuming and expensive way to solve a barking problem, could involve hiring a professional to help assess why the problem has occurred in the first place and then devise an effective plan to reverse the problem that will work for each unique situation.

Fear or Pain: another reason your dog may bark is when they are very frightened or in pain and this is usually a type of bark that sounds quite different from all the others, often being a combination of a bark and a whine, or a yelping type of noise.

This is a bark that you will want to pay close attention to, so that you can quickly respond and offer the assistance that your puppy or dog may need.

Whatever reason your dog may be barking for, always remember that this is how they communicate and *"tell"* us that they want something or are concerned, afraid, nervous or unhappy about something, and as their guardians, we humans need to pay attention.

Raised Hackles: when your dog approaches with raised hackles (the hair along the dog's back), while this can be an indication that the dog may be approaching with dominant or aggressive tendencies, it also may be an indication that he or she is excited, fearful, startled, anxious or lacks confidence.

In any of these circumstances (whether it's your dog or someone else's), it's a good idea to be respectful and keep your distance until you can assess what's really going on, because even a reactive, fearful dog can quickly turn into a biting dog, and I can tell you from personal experience that being bitten by any dog really hurts.

In a Nutshell

Learning your Dachshund's particular body language can take some time, and this Chapter will help you get started. The more you are out and about with your dog, visiting and socializing in local parks and going on walks where you will find other dogs, animals and people to observe, the more opportunity you will have to become skilled at recognizing the many subtleties of dog body language.

Paying attention to your Dachshund's verbal and body-language signals as explained above, will help you figure out what message they are trying to get across to you and this can make all the difference in preventing frustration for you both while raising a happy and well-behaved dog.

One last thought about body language and energy – check in with yourself before you walk out the door with your dog, because if you're not in the moment and have your mind on something that has nothing to do with having a successful and pleasant walk with your dog, you may be setting yourself up for trouble.

For example, if you go out the door with your dog while displaying sad, weak or confusing energy, your dog will pick up on this and become nervous or confused themselves because your energy is no longer conveying to your dog that you are their leader. This means that your energy can literally be the cause of, for instance, an uncomfortable encounter with another person walking their dog.

It's very important to keep in mind that when walking with a dog, the moment they sense that you are not completely in control, they will take this unspoken "cue" from you that being in charge has now defaulted to him or her.

You <u>never</u> want any dog to feel they must protect you from the postman, neighbor's cat or that taunting little terrier walking across the street, because if they do, you're literally out walking with a highly unpredictable, live "weapon" that could decide to go off at any moment.

Most Dachshunds can be trained to be accepting of other dogs and unknown people, if you have put in the time and properly socialized and trained them. However, should you permit your dog to get seriously out of control, you could end up with a lawsuit on your hands, and/or sky-high veterinary bills if this little companion is forced into being confrontational with a much bigger dog, and that's if you're lucky.

It's always a good idea to keep in mind that if your dog harms another dog, animal or person, the consequences could be far worse than a high vet bill. For instance, any dog that bites could face a death sentence or a ruling that they can never be seen in public unless they're wearing a muzzle.

Remember, as cute and comical as they are, Dachshunds are statistically more aggressive to both strangers and other dogs. As a result, on more than one occasion, they have made it into the top ten breeds of *"Most Aggressive Dogs"*, or *"Dogs That Bite the Most"*. The good news here is that much of how a dog's temperament will develop is closely tied to how he or she is raised by YOU.

While more than 20% display aggressive tendencies, including biting other dogs, strangers and even their owners, when you're a strong enough leader, and take the time to properly socialize and train, the Dachshund can be a happy and loving family companion.

Yes, raising a well-mannered dog with a stable and trustworthy temperament IS a big responsibility and an ongoing commitment. Give yourself the best chance and be honest, because it's far better that you fully understand what you're getting into BEFORE you and your dog may live to regret it.

Chapter 12: Training Basics for a Happy Dachshund

*"Everyone thinks they have the best dog
in the world. None of them are wrong."*
— Unknown

It's no surprise that a properly trained dog will be a much happier, safe and more secure companion that everyone enjoys being around, and that will be far less likely to develop behaviour issues later in life.

When your dog respects your leadership and there is no question that YOU are in charge, your dog can then relax and let you take the lead on training them, which is as it should be. Developing a basic training program and learning to teach your Dachshund commands and discipline is all part of starting your dog off on the right paw.

Therefore, this Chapter will focus on training basics and tips, including hand signals, as well as simple tricks that your dog will love to learn. Take heed humans, because you will be very happy you spent the time to learn everything contained in these pages.

All of our canine companions are amazing, natural athletes and because of this, no matter their size or breed, they need daily exercise to stay fit and healthy, so that they can be happily well-mannered, and part of their exercise routine includes learning at least three very important training basics, which are **"Come – Sit – Stay"**.

Every dog will require daily exercise to stay happy and healthy. They will love going for hikes, walks and little adventures with you. Your dog may even enjoy learning routines, tricks, and fun canine sports with their guardian as well as playing and socializing in a pack of other smaller dogs.

Any type of disciplined exercise you can engage in with your dog will help to exercise both their body and their mind and will burn off pent-up daily energy reserves, so that your dog will be a happy and contented companion that is relaxed and not suffering health issues from being overweight.

If you find that your dog is being a pest by chewing inappropriate items around the home or being demanding of your time, or especially unruly when visitors come to call, this is likely because their mind is not being challenged enough or their body is not being exercised often enough, or long enough each day to drain out their daily pent-up energy reserves.

A healthy, adult Dachshund will thrive when being walked several times each day and may also enjoy the challenge of being engaged in other forms of disciplined canine activity, such as Agility or Trick Training.

This affectionate and willing to learn dog is a breed of small hound that enjoys spending the majority of their time in the company of their human guardian, and when properly raised may be able to excel in many canine sports or even as a therapy dog.

Use your imagination and find out what canine sports your dog may enjoy learning. So long as you prove to him or her that you mean what you say through firm, fair direction and consistency, rather than too many treats, even this feisty little character will not feel the need to manipulate or question your authority, and will happily follow your direction.

Even at the young age of eight to ten weeks, most dogs are capable of beginning to learn anything you can teach. If you wait until they are six months old before beginning any serious training program, you could already have a stubborn problem on your hands and a disagreeable little dog that may be unwilling to heed your commands.

 The backbone of helping to develop a well-balanced and happy Dachshund is to provide them with a routine that ensures sufficient time to satisfy their particular physical and mental exercise needs, in combination with additional time to play, sniff, search and explore their world every day.

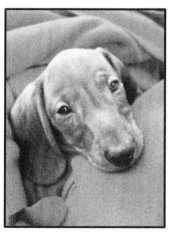 What you can teach this canine companion depends entirely upon you and the time and patience you have to devote to their education, and you never want to under estimate what incredible hidden talents your dog may have.

For instance, many of these comical and fearless weiner dogs love to swim, enjoy learning tricks, and can really excel at Agility. No matter what you decide to teach your dog, always train with patience, kindness, consistency and positive rewards.

All training sessions should be happy and fun-filled with plenty of food rewards and positive reinforcement, which will ensure that your dog is a happy, attentive student who trusts and respects you as their leader and looks forward to learning new commands, tricks and routines.

Dachshund Puppy Training Basics

First, choose a *"Discipline Sound"* that will be the same for every human family member. This will make it much easier for your Dachshund puppy to learn what they can or cannot do and will be very useful when warning or redirecting your puppy before they engage in unwanted behavior.

The best types of sounds are short and sharp, so that you and your family members can quickly say them and so that the sound will immediately get the attention of your puppy, as you want to be able to easily interrupt them when they are about to make a mistake.

It doesn't really matter what the sound is, so long as it gets your dog's attention and everyone in the family is consistent. A sound that is very effective in most cases is a simple *"UH!"* sound that is said sharply and with emphasis.

Most puppies and dogs respond immediately to this sound and if caught in the middle of doing something they are not supposed to be doing, they will quickly stop and give you their attention or back away from what they were doing.

Next, your puppy needs to learn the Three Most Important Words, which are *"Come"*, *"Sit"* and *"Stay"*. These three basic commands will ensure that your puppy remains safe in almost every circumstance.

For instance, when your puppy correctly learns the *"Come"* command, you can always quickly bring them back to you if you should see danger approaching. Also, when you teach your puppy the *"Sit"* and *"Stay"* commands, you will be further establishing your leadership role, and a puppy that understands that their human guardian is their leader will be a safe and happy follower.

Most puppies are ready to begin training at approximately 10 to 12 weeks of age (and some even earlier), so make your training sessions no more than 5 or 10 minutes (2 or 3 times a day), positive and pleasant with lots of praise and/or treats so that your puppy will be looking forward to their next session.

To help you understand the big three commands, yours truly demonstrates what the hand signals look like in the pictures below!

COME:

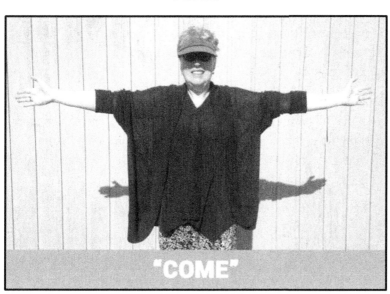

While most Dachshund puppies will be capable of learning commands and tricks at a very young age, the first and most important command you need to teach your puppy is the recall, or *"Come"* command.

- ❧ Begin the *"Come"* command inside your home.

- ❧ Go into a larger room, such as your living room area.

- ❧ Place your puppy in front of you and attach their leash or a longer line to their Martingale collar, while you back away from them a few feet.

- ❧ Say the command *"Come"* in an excited, happy voice and hold your arms open wide.

- ❧ If they do not immediately come to you, gently give a tug on the leash, so that they understand that they are supposed to move toward you.

- ❧ When they come to you, happily praise them and give a treat they really enjoy.

Once your puppy can accomplish a *"Come"* command almost every time inside your home, you can then graduate them to a nearby park or quiet outside area where you will repeat the process and where there are many more distractions. In order to keep yourself and your dog safe, he or she needs to always come to you when asked, despite whatever distractions may be nearby.

You may want to purchase an extra-long, lightweight line (25 or 50 feet), so that you are always attached to your puppy and can encourage them in the right direction should they become distracted by noises, scents and other dogs. Try to choose a time of day when there will be fewer distractions while you are training.

Once your dog always comes running when called, you will no longer need to say the "Come" word, but just show them the signal, which they will be able to see from across the park

Keep in mind that even after teaching your Dachshund the *"Come"* command, their nose may take precedence over the commands you are teaching when outdoors if an interesting scent distracts them. Always keep a young dog on leash when working in an area where they can easily run off in pursuit of an intriguing scent.

SIT:

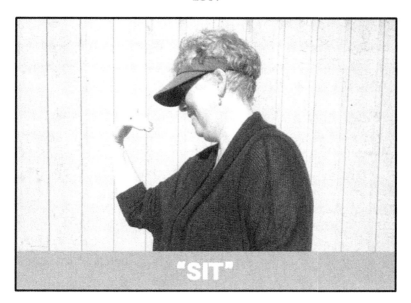

The "Sit" and "*Stay*" commands are both easy commands to teach that will help to keep your puppy safe and out of danger in almost every circumstance. Find a quiet time to teach these commands when your puppy is not overly tired.

* Ask your puppy to "Sit" and if they do not yet understand the command, show them what you mean by gently squeezing with your thumb and middle finger the area across the back that joins with their back legs.

* Do NOT just push them down into a sit, as this can cause damage to their back or joints.

* When they sit, give them a treat and praise them.

* When you say the word "Sit", at the same time show them the hand signal for this command.

* While you can use any hand signal, the universal hand signal for "Sit" is right arm (palm open facing upward) parallel to the floor, and then raising your arm while bending at the elbow toward your right shoulder.

❧ Once your dog is sitting reliably for you, remove the verbal "Sit" and replace it with the hand signal.

Every time you take your dog out for a walk, which is often a cause of excitement, get into the habit of asking them to sit quietly and patiently at every stage of your walk.

For instance, ask your dog to sit and patiently wait while you put on their leash, while you put on your shoes or jacket, after you approach the door, after you are on the other side of the door, while you lock the door, every time you arrive at a street intersection or crosswalk, every time you stop during your walk to speak to a neighbor, greet a friend or admire the view, etc., and do this all in reverse when heading back home.

When you persist with the *"Sit"* training, it will soon become automatic for your dog to calmly sit every time you stop walking.

When you ask your dog to sit for you, they are learning several things all at once; that they must remain calm while paying attention to you, that you are the boss, that they must look to you for direction and that they must respect you as their leader.

Keep in mind that a sitting puppy is much easier to control than one standing at the alert, ready to bolt out the door or jump on someone. As well, because the action of sitting helps to calm the mind of an excited puppy (or dog), teaching your puppy the *"Sit"* command is a very important part of their daily interactions with your family members as well as people you may meet when out on a walk.

When you ask your puppy to *"Sit"* before you interact in any way with them, before you go out, before you feed them, etc., you are helping to quiet their mind, while teaching them to look to you for direction, and at the same time making it more difficult for them to jump, lunge or disappear out a door.

STAY:

"STAY"

* Once your puppy can reliably "Sit", say the word "Stay" (with authority in your voice) and hold your outstretched arm, palm open toward their head while backing away a few steps.

* If they try to follow, calmly say "No" and put them back into "Sit".

* Give a treat and then say again, "Stay" with the hand signal and back away a few steps.

* Practice these three basic "Come", "Sit", "Stay" commands everywhere you go, and use the "Sit" command as much as you can to ensure its success rate.

As your puppy gets older, and their attention span increases, you will be able to train for longer periods of time and introduce more complicated routines. This is a very smart dog that can easily learn many hand signals.

Hand Signals

It's really important to use the hand signals that go along with the verbal commands during training, so that once your Dachshund learns both, you can remove the verbal commands in favor of just hand signals.

Hand signal training is by far the most useful and efficient training method for your dog. All too often we inundate our canine companions with a great deal of chatter and noise that they really don't understand, but because they are so willing to be part of our world, they soon learn the meaning of many words.

Contrary to what some people might think, the first language of a Dachshund (or any dog) is a combination of sensing energy and watching body language, which requires no spoken word or sound.

Therefore, when we humans take the time to teach our dog hand signals for all their basic commands, we are communicating with them at a level they instinctively understand, plus we are helping them to become a focused follower, as they must watch us in order to understand what is required of them.

Simple Tricks

When teaching your dog tricks, in order to give him or her extra incentive, find a treat that they really like and give the treat as a positive reward, which will help solidify a good performance.

Most dogs will be extra attentive during training sessions when they know that they will be rewarded with their favorite treats – especially this dog, who will usually have a healthy appetite.

If your puppy is less than six months old when you begin teaching them tricks, keep your training sessions short (no more than 5 or 10 minutes) and fun. As they become adults, you can extend your sessions, as they will be able to maintain their focus for longer periods of time.

SHAKE A PAW:

Who doesn't love a well-trained dog that knows how to shake a paw? This is one of the easiest tricks to teach your dog.

- ❧ Find a quiet place to practice, without noisy distractions or other pets, and stand or sit in front of your dog.

- ❧ Place them in the sitting position and have a treat in your left hand.

- ❧ Say the command "Shake" while putting your right hand behind their left or right paw and pulling the paw gently toward yourself until you are holding their paw in your hand.

- ❧ Immediately praise them and give them their favorite treat.

- ❧ Most smart and willing dogs will learn the "Shake" trick quite quickly, and very soon, once you put out your hand, your dog will immediately lift their paw and put it into your hand, without your assistance or any verbal cue.

Practice every day until they are 100% reliable with this trick, and then it will be time to add another trick to their repertoire.

Most dogs are naturally either right or left pawed. If you know which paw your dog favors, ask them to shake this paw.

ROLL OVER:

Step #1   Step #2   Step #3

"Roll Over" (this is circular motion)

You will find that just as your dog is naturally either right or left pawed, they will also naturally want to roll either to the right or the left side. Take advantage of this by asking your dog to roll to the side they naturally prefer.

- ❧ Sit with your dog on the floor and put them in a lie down position.

- ❧ Hold a treat in your hand and place it close to their nose without allowing them to grab it.

- ❧ While they are in the lying position, move the treat to the right or left side of their head (the nose will follow the treat), so that they have to roll over to get to it.

- ❧ You will very quickly see which side they want to naturally roll to, and once you see this, move the treat to this side.

* When they roll over to this side, immediately give them the treat and praise them.

* You can say the verbal cue "Over" while you demonstrate the hand signal motion (moving your right hand in a circular motion) or moving the treat from one side of their head to the other with a half circle motion.

SIT PRETTY:

While this trick is a little more complicated, and most dogs pick up on it very quickly, remember that every dog is different so always exercise patience.

* Find a quiet space with few distractions and sit or stand in front of your dog and ask them to "Sit".

* Have a treat nearby (on a countertop or table) and when they sit, use both of your hands to lift up their front paws into the sitting pretty position, while saying the command "Sit Pretty".

* Help them balance in this position, while you praise them and give them the treat.

🐾 Once your dog can perform the balancing part of the trick quite easily without your help, sit or stand in front of your dog while asking them to "Sit Pretty".

🐾 Holding the treat above their head at the level of their nose would be when they sit pretty.

🐾 If they attempt to stand on their back legs to get the treat, you may be holding the treat too high, which will encourage them to stand on their back legs to reach it. Go back to the first step and put them back into the "Sit" position and again lift their paws while their backside remains on the floor.

🐾 After they learn the trick on verbal command, try saying the verbal cue while demonstrating the hand signal: holding your straight arm, fully extended, over your dog's head with a closed fist (pictured).

🐾 Make this a fun and entertaining time for both of you and practice a few times every day until they can "Sit Pretty" on hand signal command every time you ask.

A smart young puppy should be able to easily learn these basic tricks before they are six months old and when you are patient and make your training sessions short and fun for your dog, they will be eager to learn so much more.

Crate Training

The best method for housetraining your dog is called crate training. Basically, you give your puppy many opportunities to do his business outside, so he isn't tempted to do it inside.

During times when you cannot keep a constant watch on your puppy (such as when you're making dinner or sleeping), you put him or her in their crate so they do not have an accident. As long as you use the crate for this purpose and you help your puppy form a positive association with the crate, he will not mind being in it. Just do not use it as a form of punishment!

So, how exactly do you go about house training your puppy? Here's a step-by-step guide:

1. Choose a certain part of your yard where you want your dog to go.
2. Take your puppy outside every hour or so -- directly to the chosen spot every time.
3. When you take your puppy out, say "Go pee" as soon as you set him or her down in that area.
4. Wait for your puppy to do his business – and the moment they do, immediately praise them in an excited voice and give a small treat as a reward.
5. If your puppy does not have to go, take them back inside instead of letting him wander around.
6. When you are at home, keep a close eye on your puppy and confine them to whatever room you are in.

7. Watch your dog for signs that he or she has to go and take them outside immediately if they start to sniff the ground, walk in circles, or squat.
8. During times when you cannot physically watch your puppy, put him or her in their crate to reduce the risk of an accident – do not keep any food or water in the crate with them.
9. Let your puppy go outside to relieve his or herself immediately before putting them in the crate and also immediately after releasing them. You should also take your puppy outside shortly after a meal or when they wake up from a nap.

10. Take away your puppy's food and water about an hour before bedtime until they are able to go the whole night without an accident.

When you first bring your puppy home, you shouldn't expect him or her to be able to hold their bladder or bowels for more than an hour or two. Even so, you should start crate training right away so they learn good habits from an early age. As they get older, they will be able to wait longer before needing a bathroom break – about one hour for each month of age.

Adult Training

This is a dog that will thrive so long as they are getting to spend fun time close to their human. Therefore, in order to ensure a happy and healthy dog that will not develop behaviour issues out of boredom or laziness, make sure that you get your dog involved in some fun activity, such as Advanced Obedience, Trick Training, or perhaps Barn Hunt, Earth Dog or Field Trials that will appeal to their hunting history.

When your dog is a full-grown adult (approximately two years of age), you will definitely want to begin more complicated or advanced training sessions.

When you have the desire and patience, you may be surprised at how many commands, tricks, routines or canine sports you can teach a happy, willing Dachshund who trusts and respects their human guardian.

For instance, you may wish to teach your adult dog more advanced tricks, such as opposite sided paw shakes or rollovers, which are more difficult than you might expect and which the smart Dachshund is definitely capable of learning.

If you and your dog are really enjoying learning new tricks or routines together, consider teaching them a series of hand signals, such as *"Commando crawl"*, *"Speak"* or *"Jump through the human hoop"*, or perhaps get them certified as a therapy dog so they can brighten the days of those who must spend time in hospitals and care facilities.

Teaching your dog tricks and routines builds trust and respect, is fun for both of you, and a healthy way to exercise both your dog's mind and body, which will result in a happy, contented and well-behaved companion.

Over-Exercising

Be especially careful about over-exercising your Dachshund when it's warm out and when they are really young (as their muscles and bones are not yet fully developed), because like humans, dogs can also collapse from heat stroke. Keep in mind that this dog may have a very strong prey drive and chasing that fast moving ball may be so exciting to him or her that they may not know when to quit.

Playtime

Every dog needs some down time or regular playtime each day, and while every dog will be different with respect to what types of games they may enjoy, most will really love any game involving retrieving a ball or soft toy.

The smart Dachshund may also be a very excited participant in a fun game of *"Search"*, where you ask your dog to *"Sit/Stay"* while you hide a favorite treat that they then have to use their nose to find.

To begin teaching the "Search" game, first time ask your dog to sit/stay while you slowly back away and place a treat where they can actually still see it. Return to where they are in their sit/stay and say, "OK! Search!" and point to where you just placed the treat. Each time you play this game, you can place the treat farther and farther away and completely out of their sight before you release them to "Search!"

After a disciplined walk with your dog, they will also enjoy being given the opportunity for some off-leash freedom to really stretch out by running free to play and socialize with other similar-sized dogs at the local dog park.

In a Nutshell

Taking the time to teach your dog basic rules and boundaries, plus simple or complex tricks, will keep them both mentally and physically healthy and happy and you will raise a well-behaved dog that is a joy to be around.

The Dachshund will usually be a very smart, and willing to please little dog. In order to ensure a healthy, happy and contented dog that is not overweight and will not develop behavior issues out of boredom or neglect, you must take the time to involve them in daily moderate to high amounts of exercise; that can include different activities, such as interesting canine sports where they get to develop their unique skills.

Chapter 13: What If You Slip Up?

"Dogs got personality.
Personality goes a long way."
— Quentin Tarantino

All the information, suggestions, tips and advice given in this book is the result of more than 40 years experience helping humans positively and effectively interact with the canine world.

If you take all that is written on these pages to heart, and regularly and consistently apply them, your Dachshund will grow up to be a happy family member that will not have to suffer from any behavioral issues.

However, if your lifestyle drastically changes, you forget to exercise your dog, keep on top of basic or advanced training, or you slip up for any number of reasons, problems may inevitably occur.

For instance, you may end up becoming too busy or distracted with your human life to provide your canine companion with what he or she needs on a daily basis to be a happy and fulfilled member of your family.

Realistically, there may be any number of other reasons why you don't consistently apply the information given here, and the following is an outline of just a few of the more common behavioral issues that may occur, with some tips that may help you get back on track.

When reading the following pages, please keep in mind that a specific behavioral problem is usually the result of many different possibilities or circumstances that have taken place between the human individual or family and the particular dog.

This means that properly addressing a specific unwanted behavior often needs the assistance of a professional with a personal approach, who can ask the right questions to determine how the unwanted behavior occurred, because it's often not what you may have initially thought.

Therefore, to generically outline possible ways to reverse an unwanted behavior will be a guessing game, because without knowing the circumstances of the guardian and their family, and understanding the situation that triggered the unwanted behavior, I can only make my best guess based on previous experience with similar problems.

As an example, there might be many reasons why the Dachshund in question is chewing the tassels on your Persian rug. For instance, this could be because they:

- are hungry

- are teething

- have a taste for wool

- think the tassels are a toy

- are a super high energy dog

- 🐾 are left alone and are bored

- 🐾 haven't been given appropriate toys to chew

- 🐾 have not been taught rules and what is appropriate

- 🐾 need a guardian with stronger leadership energy

- 🐾 are under-exercised

- 🐾 are over-stimulated

As you can see, it's possible for almost endless scenarios and reasons why a dog may develop a particular behavioral issue.

Therefore, please understand that without close observation and much more information explaining a particular situation, the following few common behavioral problems and the suggestions for alleviating them, will be my best guess.

Chewing Inappropriate Items
[Re-visit *"Distraction and Replacement"* in Chapter 10]

If your puppy or dog is chewing the carpet, your fingers, the legs of the coffee table, or any other inappropriate item(s) that are not dog toys, rather than getting upset with your dog, you need to train yourself to be much more vigilant, and then distract and replace.

First make sure that all the chewing is not just because the puppy is teething. Have compassion because teething is painful for the puppy and they must chew to help alleviate the pain while those adult teeth are growing in.

Always make sure your puppy has plenty of chew toys and to help with the teething pain, give your puppy an old T-towel soaked in water, tied in knots and frozen in the freezer as a chew toy.

When your Dachshund is a little older, already has pushed through their adult set of teeth and has decided, for instance, that the legs on your coffee table are good chew toys, it is possible that you:

🐾 are not paying attention and taking the time to make sure your dog receives enough daily exercise, and/or,

🐾 are not teaching your dog what is, and what is not, appropriate for chewing by saying a firm and convincing "No", replacing the table leg with a toy they are allowed to chew, and praising them when they've got the right thing between their teeth.

Being Fearful of Loud Noises
[Re-visit *"Fear of Loud Noises"* in Chapter 10]

If you have raised a dog that has a fear of loud, popping noises, perhaps you haven't taken the time to read this information and apply the suggestions outlined, so read it now and practice until your dog loses or at least diminishes their fear.

Excessive Excitement When Friends Visit
[Re-visit *"Chapter 3: Overview of the Happy Dachshund"* and *"Chapter 12: Training Basics for a Happy Dachshund"*]

Make sure that you begin to teach an excitable young Dachshund to be a calm follower as soon as you bring him or her home.

Always ignore an excited dog and do <u>not</u> touch them until they are calm and relaxed, otherwise you will inadvertently teach them that it is acceptable behavior for them to be excited every time they see a human.

If they are overly excited when friends come to visit, stand between your dog and your friends, and create some space by pointing away and firmly telling your dog, *"GO"*, and also ask your friends to ignore him or her.

Also, if you've been properly training your puppy or dog, you will have taught them to *"Sit"* on command, and a sitting dog is much more relaxed and easier to control.

Acting Aggressively on a Walk
[Re-visit *"Chapter 12: Training Basics for a Happy Dachshund"*]

Make sure that your dog is walking at your side without pulling on the leash when you are out for a walk.

When you train your dog to walk beside you, this "tells" them that YOU are their leader and in charge of every situation, which means they will be much less likely to act out or attempt to "protect" you from outside stimuli. If they DO try, immediately give a sharp tug on that Martingale collar along with a strong *"NO!"* to remind them who is the boss.

Pulling When on Leash
[Re-visit *"The Martingale Collar"* in Chapter 10]

If your dog is pulling on leash, chances are high that he or she is not wearing the proper training collar and you have not taken the time to teach them to quietly walk at your side.

Buy your dog a Martingale collar, properly adjust it, and then the next time they try to pull ahead of you, give a sharp snap to this collar (toward yourself) and firmly say the word *"Heel"*.

Repeating this process until your dog understands can take a few minutes or even several days, as each dog is different – be consistent and persistent until your dog gets it.

Also, turning circles and changing directions suddenly when on a leash walk will quickly help to teach your dog their proper walking position, because if they are ahead of you they are going to be stepped on or walked into.

Stealing Food or Raiding the Garbage Can

[Re-visit *"Ideal Living Conditions for a Happy Dachshund"* in Chapter 6]

Make sure you absolutely understand that while the Dachshund may be a particularly food motivated breed, if given the opportunity and the food is enticing enough, any dog will steal food. This means that in order to avoid this possibility, you must be a vigilant guardian and make sure that you never leave any food they should not eat unattended or where they can reach it.

Not Obeying Commands

[Re-visit *"Chapter 12: Training Basics for a Happy Dachshund"*]

A well-trained Dachshund is one that obeys the basic *"Come/Sit/Stay"* commands. If your dog is not obeying your commands, you have not taken the time to properly train them, or you are too weak a leader, with the result being that he or she will take a stubborn attitude, they will ignore you and they will not respect you as their leader. Get to work right away, step up your energy to ensure you are a strong enough leader for this fearless little hound, and train your dog so that everyone will be happy.

> **TIP**
> *We all have our off days, so don't get down on yourself if you occasionally slip up and are not being as vigilant, strong and confident a leader as you need to be with this dog's basic and/or advanced training and daily maintaining of rules and boundaries.*

In a Nutshell

We humans will always have days when we are not as vigilant as we need to be, which means that we will inevitably "slip up" sometimes when raising our fur friends.

What you need to remember is that it's not the end of the world, because there is always a solution, and often simply re-reading the relevant chapters in this book can quickly and easily get you back on track to raising a happy and well-behaved Dachshund that is a pleasure to be around.

Also, know that the familiar expression *"You can't teach an old dog new tricks"* is totally false. It doesn't matter what age a particular dog may be, because with the right knowledge, patience and persistence, you absolutely CAN teach a dog of any age new tricks.

Chapter 14: Surprise Bonus Chapter

*"Dogs have a way of finding the people
who need them, and filling an emptiness
we didn't ever know we had."*
— Thom Jones

If you thought that you had reached the end of this book, well surprise, not quite yet, as I'd like to leave you with some canine wisdom and a short, funny, true story.

Happy Dachshund Question and Answer (Q&A) section

The following Question and Answer (Q&A) section is written from the dog's perspective, and although you may find it amusing, there are also valuable human lessons to be learned, if anyone is paying attention.

First, let me set the scene for the following situations:

This is a young, busy family, consisting of Mom and Dad, who work at home, one 12-year-old girl, and one 14-year-old boy, who share their lives with a neutered, 2-year-old dog named Harvey. They all live together in a large house with a medium-sized, fenced yard out the back.

The following questions, asked by various members of the family, are directed to the dog, and answered by the dog, as if the dog could talk like their humans.

Each question that the dog answers is followed by a short synopsis of the "lesson" we humans can learn from these various interactions.

Mom: **"Oh No! Why did you pee on the floor?"**

Harvey: *"Ah, maybe because I drank a bowl of water after my dinner, and you forgot to let me out before everyone left for that baseball game, and I just couldn't hold it any longer."*

Lesson: Humans often lead very busy lives, and in order to ensure their dog remains happy, they still need to always pay attention and put their canine friend's habits and needs ahead of their own.

Girl: **"Yuckeeee! Harvey, why do you smell like dog poo?"**

Harvey: *"Could it be because, as much as I tried to tiptoe through those piles of doggy doo in the back yard, that as far as I'm concerned smell much better than tulips, I was chasing a squirrel and accidentally stepped in one."*

"Can't take my dog?! But I don't even know HOW to run without my dog!"

Lesson: Humans with convenient back yard doggy bathrooms often forget to be vigilant about picking up the yard. This is not only a smelly bad habit that busy (or lazy) guardians are guilty of, it's also a considerable health hazard that attracts rats.

Boy: **"What's wrong, Harvey? You like to fetch — go get that ball!"**

Harvey: *"Yes, I like to fetch, but it's hot out here, and I'm getting exhausted."*

Lesson: Sometimes we humans that share our lives with dogs tend to forget that the temperature of the day that doesn't seem extreme to us, can quickly be too much for a dog that is running back and forth fetching a ball. We also forget that many dogs, despite their discomfort, may continue to fetch that ball even though they may be about to collapse from heat exhaustion.

Dad: **"What happened in here, Harvey! You've made a huge mess and knocked over all these boxes I had neatly stacked in the carport! What's wrong with you?"**

Harvey: *"Wait a minute - nothing wrong with me! There was a squirrel in here eating through the boxes and I was just trying to protect the home. I finally got rid of him, and he won't be coming back, so don't blame me for that irritating squirrel's antics. You should be thanking me."*

Lesson: Often we tend to quickly blame our canine friends when a mess is created for which there seems to be no explanation. We need to first think beyond simply blaming the dog for unexplained disarray, as there is often a good explanation that, in most cases, exonerates your canine companion.

Mom: **"Harvey! What have you done? I left a plate of butter on the coffee table. Did you eat it?"**

Harvey: *"Thanks for leaving that out for me. It tasted really good and I sure enjoyed it at the time, but now I'm feeling a little under the weather."*

Lesson: Many of our canine companions don't know when to stop when it comes to filling their stomach. Therefore, if you have one of these dogs with an endless appetite for anything remotely resembling food, you need to be vigilant about never leaving kitchen food, garbage or anything edible where they can reach it.

Boy: **"You bad, bad dog, Harvey! You've chewed the laces off my expensive tennis shoes."**

Harvey: *"What's the big stink about? You gave me your old shoes to play with, and now you're mad at me? Someone's confused."*

Lesson: Think about what you allow your canine friend to play with, because giving them old discarded shoes, socks or other articles of clothing, etc., to play with causes confusion in the canine mind when you get mad if they decide to chew your new shoes.

Girl: **"You're covering my bed in mud, Harvey! Get out!"**

Harvey: *"Forget it! You let me sleep in your bed when I was a puppy, so move over and let me in."*

Lesson: If you'd rather not share your bed with a dog that could have just raced through a mud puddle, don't make the mistake of allowing them to sleep with you when they're a cute and much smaller cuddly puppy. If you do, it's unfair to blame your canine companion for wanting to continue this habit that you literally taught them.

Dad: **"Are you kidding me, Harvey! Where's the hot dog I left on the picnic table!"**

Harvey: *"I saved it from a circling crow and ate it while you were getting a beer. It was delicious - got any more?"*

Lesson: Dogs are carnivorous and no matter their size, whether a tiny Dachshund or a large Mastiff, if given the opportunity, their desire to eat meat is a strong instinct they cannot ignore. If you leave meat unattended, and your dog eats it, too bad stupid human - don't blame your canine companion.

Moral of the Q&A section

Always DO pay attention to what your dog is trying to tell you, because (in addition to the above), there are so many other lessons we humans can learn from our beloved canine companions. Watching out and learning these lessons, and appropriately acting upon them, will help you to raise a Happy Dachshund that will never have to experience unwanted behaviors.

There are so many lessons we humans can learn from our beloved canine companions IF we are paying attention.

Happy Dachshund True Story

Before we close this Chapter, I hope you will enjoy the following true short story:

Ozzy's New Tiles

I was dog-sitting Ozzy for clients of mine who had just recently installed a new tile entranceway in their home where previously there had been carpet tiles. The owners warned me that they were having a *"little problem"* getting Ozzy used to the new, shiny and quite slippery tiles and I told them not to worry about it, as I presumed this was a minor issue.

However, I soon found out that the joke was on me, because once I had delivered Ozzy's owners to the airport and I returned to the home with

Ozzy on leash at my side and I opened the front door, I was brought to a sudden abrupt halt when Ozzy refused to enter the house.

Ozzy stopped so suddenly that all the groceries I was carrying became airborne and ended up strewn across the floor while it felt like I had suddenly become attached to a wriggling fire hydrant. OK, so much for the *"little"* problem Ozzy was having with the new flooring because he flatly refused to put even one paw on those shiny new tiles.

Thank goodness it was a pleasant summer day because now was the time to start working out Ozzy's fear of shiny surfaces and this meant keeping the front door open.

I tied Ozzy's leash to the railing near the door, rescued my groceries from the tiled floor, found some of Ozzy's favorite treats, and returned to untie Ozzy while I showed him I had something he wanted. He was immediately interested in the treats and started to follow me into the house only to abruptly stop at the door.

I went inside a couple of feet and sat down with his treats on the tiled surface, holding my hand out to offer him one. He stretched as far as he could without stepping on the tiles trying to get to the treats he really wanted, while I kept calmly encouraging him to move forward.

Finally, after several failed attempts to get him to put a paw on the dreaded tile surface, he completely flattened himself onto his belly and used his legs like a frog to *"swim"* his way across the tiles to get the treats I was offering.

This was definitely one of the funniest things I had ever seen a dog do, but I had to be careful not to laugh because he needed me to be his strong and confident leader, so I stifled my laughter and praised him for being so brave.

So now here was Ozzy flat on his belly in the middle of the shiny tile surface with his beloved carpeting about ten slippery tiles away. I stood up and moved farther into the house onto the carpeted area, still encouraging him to come and get his favorite treats.

He looked up at me with those big pleading eyes that seemed to say *"help me out of this predicament"*, and all I could do was talk softly and confidently to him, pretending everything was just fine as I asked him to come and get his treats.

After a couple of minutes, Ozzy decided that the only way to get what he wanted was to *"swim"* a little farther and he flailed with his front paws and kicked with his back feet like a frog until he made his way onto the carpet, where he immediately bounded into life.

Stifling my laughter, I immediately praised and petted him, gave him several of his favorite treats, and all was now right in Ozzy's world, until it came time to go out for a lunchtime walk around the block.

I hitched up Ozzy's leash to his Martingale collar and started to walk toward the front door, which involved crossing over the tiled entranceway, hoping he would forget about his fear, but as soon as we reached the edge of the carpet, he immediately put the brakes on.

I stopped with him, keeping some forward tension on his leash, as I offered him a treat if he would just take one step onto the tiles. Instead, he immediately dropped onto his belly again, like a penguin about to slide down a snow bank, and started pushing himself across the tiles to get to the treat I was offering.

Such a sight he was and so determined to get his treat without having to walk – you had to give him credit for his amazing ingenuity.

When he got to my outstretched hand and gobbled down his treat, I gently picked him up and placed his feet onto the dreaded tiles and again encouraged him to walk toward me. This time, although he remained crouched low, he gingerly attempted his first step, and then another and another until you could actually see a light bulb go off in his little doggy brain when he realized that the smooth surface of the tiles was indeed safe to walk on.

I happily praised him for his bravery and gave him another treat, and then a few more times in and out the door and although he would slightly hesitate when stepping onto the tiles, and stoop down to sniff them, within three days of practicing our little routine, the dreaded slippery tile flooring was no longer a problem for this comical little character.

When his owners returned from their holiday, you can imagine how happy they were to know that they no longer had to carry Ozzy across their entranceway.

Lesson to learn: **No matter the age of your dog, and how much you may have socialized them, when you change something in their world, they can become nervous, scared and traumatized. The only way to work through this is with much patience and understanding, coupled with persistent calm energy, and of course, favorite treats.**

Chapter 15: Conclusion and Reviews

"Once you have a wonderful dog,
a life without one is a life diminished."
— Dean Koontz

This book is written to help anyone thinking of sharing their life with the playful and affectionate Dachshund, to first understand whether or not they truly have the time, energy and lifestyle that would be compatible with raising a healthy and happy dog.

Once it's been decided that the smart, loving and loyal Dachshund is the right breed to share your life with, the purpose of this book is to help you understand how to properly care for them. This will include socializing, training and providing this dog with adequate physical and mental daily exercise, the best food, and a safe environment, so that this dog can live the longest and most contented life possible.

There are already plenty of books written, and many different trainers and opinions concerning how to correct a dog that may be suffering from any number of behavioral issues.

However, to my knowledge, there are no breed-specific books outlining how most, if not all, behavioral issues are unknowingly created by the dog's human guardian. Therefore, this breed-specific book stands out from all other current publications, because it:

❧ highlights that almost all problems, both mentally and physically, are a direct result of ignorance or unwillingness on the part of the human guardian to learn what their dog truly needs.

❧ describes in detail what the human guardian needs to understand and commit to doing on a daily basis in order to match the Dachshund's needs, so that they can raise a happy, healthy and well-behaved dog that never has to experience behavioral issues.

There is much knowledge for this breed contained within the pages of this book that has been gained over some 40 years working with dogs. This information will help anyone serious about raising a happy Dachshund, so that they can easily implement all the practical tips of this book without having to hire a professional to help them correct any sort of future behavioral problems.

In a nutshell, this book contains all you need to raise a Happy Dachshund that will never have to experience unwanted behaviors or join the ranks of the "aggressive and noisy small dog". When you give your dog what he or she needs to be happy, the outcome for everyone will inevitably be just that – Happy!

What Past Clients Have to Say

The following are a few happy reviews from some of my past dog whispering clients, who did the work required to turn their Dachshund into a happy and well-behaved companion. I have taught these clients how to apply some of the tips and techniques described in this book (such as how to establish yourself as the pack leader) and they easily managed to get back on track to raising a happy and well-behaved companion.

Thus, rather than taking my word for the effectiveness of the methods contained in this book, perhaps you would prefer to take my clients' word!!

> *"Thank you for your report and teaching me to be a pack leader … this has worked remarkably as Drew and Sammy have responded well beyond my expectations… Drew is very calm and relaxed and our walks are now very enjoyable…*
>
> *I want you to know that I really appreciate your help… Results have been spectacular and both dogs have evolved into superheroes and have accepted me as their pack leader and respond positively…"*
> ~ Klaus, Drew, Sammy & Max the Cat

> *"I just wanted to thank you again for our lesson today. You really are amazing with dogs. Tim and I learned so much from you, it's really neat to see the difference it makes in the dogs when you take control…"*
> ~ Morgan, Tim, Grizzly, Bella & Bear

> *"I was at the point I was ready to give Jake away because I was so concerned about how he reacted every time someone came to the door. It was really embarrassing! Honestly, within three hours of Asia being here, Jake was a different dog. We learned how to become the pack leader and control him…"*
> ~ Sharon, Mike & Jake

> *"My partner and I and our dog Rollo recently moved to Victoria from up north. Rollo, unused to city life and walking on a leash, was nervous and reactive around other dogs. Asia showed us how we need to behave so he could relax. After just one session the difference was very impressive – walks have become relaxing and enjoyable again – for all of us…"*
> ~ Tim, Mary & Rollo

> *"Thank you for helping me become the guardian that Ida needs. She was a good dog to start with, now she is an incredible dog. She walks well on lead, stays in my unfenced yard, and comes*

when called. I am often complimented on what a well-behaved dog I have. Thanks for making it all happen..."
~ Kristiane & Ida

Published by Worldwide Information Publishing 2020

Copyright and Trademarks: This publication is Copyrighted 2020 by Worldwide Information Publishing. All products, publications, software and services mentioned and recommended in this publication are protected by trademarks. In such instance, all trademarks & copyright belong to the respective owners. All rights reserved.

No part of this book may be reproduced or transferred in any form or by any means, graphic, electronic, or mechanical, including photocopying, recording, taping, or by any information storage retrieval system, without the written permission of the authors. Pictures used in this book are either royalty free pictures bought from stock-photo websites or have the source mentioned underneath the picture.

Disclaimer and Legal Notice: This product is not legal or medical advice and should not be interpreted in that manner. You need to do your own due-diligence to determine if the content of this product is right for you. The authors and the affiliates of this product are not liable for any damages or losses associated with the content in this product.

While every attempt has been made to verify the information shared in this publication, neither the author nor the affiliates assume any responsibility for errors, omissions or contrary interpretation of the subject matter herein. Any perceived slights to any specific person(s) or organization(s) are purely unintentional. We have no control over the nature, content and availability of the web sites listed in this book.

The accuracy and completeness of information provided herein and opinions stated herein are not guaranteed or warranted to produce any particular results, and the advice and strategies, contained herein may not be suitable for every individual. The authors shall not be liable for any loss incurred as a consequence of the use and application, directly or indirectly, of any information presented in this work. This publication is designed to provide information in regard to the subject matter covered.

The information included in this book has been compiled to give an overview of the subject and detail some of the symptoms, treatments etc. that are available. It is not intended to give medical advice. For a firm diagnosis of any health condition, and for a treatment plan suitable for you and your dog, you should consult your veterinarian or consultant.

The writers of this book and the publisher are not responsible for any damages or negative consequences that may arise as a result of following any of the treatments or methods highlighted in this book.

Printed in Great Britain
by Amazon

20928375R00119